D0071040

Practical Illustrated Histology

N. A. Ratcliffe

Department of Zoology
University College of Swansea

P. J. Llewellyn

Department of Zoology
University College of Swansea

Macmillan Publishing Co., Inc.
New York

Copyright © 1982, N. A. Ratcliffe and P. J. Llewellyn

Printed in Hong Kong

All rights reserved. No part of this book may be reproduced or
transmitted in any form or by any means, electronic or mechanical,
including photocopying, recording, or any information storage and
retrieval system, without permission in writing from the Publisher.

Macmillan Publishing Co., Inc.
866 Third Avenue, New York, New York 10022

ISBN: 0-02-398560-7

Photographs and text by N. A. Ratcliffe
Line illustrations by P. J. Llewellyn

Printing: 1 2 3 4 5 6 7 8   Year: 2 3 4 5 6 7 8 9 0

The paperback edition of this book is sold subject to the condition that it shall not, by way of trade
or otherwise, be lent, resold, hired out, or otherwise circulated without the publisher's prior consent
in any form of binding or cover other than that in which it is published and without a similar
condition including this condition being imposed on the subsequent purchaser.

Practical Illustrated Histology

Contents

Preface

Practical Illustrated Histology is designed to assist the student in the laboratory with the identification and understanding of histological sections. To this end, low-, medium- and high-power photomicrographs of most mammalian tissues are presented and also accurate and clearly labelled drawings together with lists of characteristic features. The micrographs are thus not covered in distractive and obscure labelling while the drawings allow some licence for clarification of indistinct features. The importance of the interrelationship of structure with function is also emphasised throughout by the listing of both tissue characteristics and functions, and by means of brief synopses, of basic physiology and morphology, at the beginning of each chapter.

This book is written primarily for students new to histology at school and college levels and, in order briefly to introduce the subject to the beginner, the first chapter contains basic information on the cell, methods of microscopy, resolution, cell morphology and ultrastructure.

Practical Illustrated Histology, however, is not aimed at replacing the more advanced theoretical texts but, with its synopses and diagrams of the main systems of the body, together with the clearly labelled drawings and summaries of characteristic features and functions, it should prove most useful not only as an introductory manual but also for both revision and reference purposes.

Additional features which underline the value of the book at the bench level are the inclusion of step-by-step practical schedules for tissue processing and staining. Detailed instructions are given for the commonly used haematoxylin and eosin technique and also for the more advanced staining methods which have been employed in the book. Advice is also provided on microtomy, the interpretation and drawing of histological sections and on microscope calibration and micrometry.

During the preparation of this book, innumerable friends and colleagues have generously assisted me by providing material and/or advice and I wish to thank, in particular, Dr M. S. Berry, Dr P. F. Brain, Mr R. G. Elias, Mr P. Fleetwood, Mr M. R. Fordy, Mrs M. Griffiths, Dr P. Makings, Dr A. F. Rowley and Mr I. Tew, all of whom are past or present members of the Department of Zoology, University College of Swansea, Mrs P. A. Green of Philip Harris Biological Ltd, and Dr J. G. Richards of Hoffman–La Roche & Co. Ltd. I am also indebted to Miss B. Jones, Mrs M. Thomas, Miss L. Millett and Mrs P. Llewellyn for typing the manuscript.

Finally, Paul Llewellyn and myself wish to dedicate this book to our respective wives, Carolyn and Pauline, for their magnificent support during the years involved in its preparation.

Swansea, 1981   N.A.R.

1 The Cell — Structure and Methods of Observation

The body is composed of small, membrane-bound units of protoplasm called cells. Each cell can usually carry out all of the processes, such as respiration, excretion and division, necessary for the maintenance of life. Cells vary enormously in size from 5–8 µm (red blood cells) to several hundred micrometres in diameter (egg cells), although most fall within the 5–30 µm range. Cells are also of many diverse forms, with their shape often reflecting their function. Thus, nerve cells tend to be elongated for the transmission of messages along their cytoplasmic pro-

cesses. Within the body, like cells are usually grouped together to form various sorts of tissues. These tissues, however, are rarely composed of just one cell type, although one kind of cell usually predominates.

The protoplasm of the cell is composed of a single, round nucleus surrounded by a mass of protoplasm, termed the cytoplasm. The nucleus contains the hereditary material, the genes, in the deoxyribonucleic acid of the chromosomes, whereas the cytoplasm encloses the various organelles responsible for the day-to-day life

Fig. 1.1.(a)   Light microscope

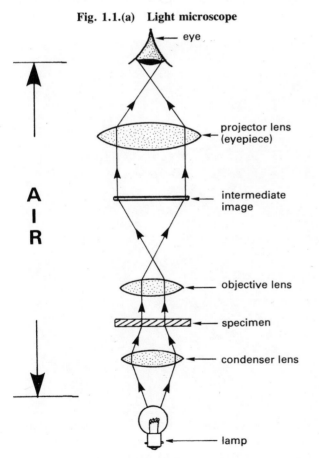

Fig. 1.1.(b)   Electron microscope

Fig. 1.1.   Diagram showing much-simplified layouts of (a) light microscope and (b) electron microscope

processes. Frequent interchanges of nutrients and information do, however, occur between the nucleus and cytoplasm.

Various methods of observation of cell structure have been developed including bright-field, phase-contrast and electron microscopy.

1.1   BRIGHT-FIELD MICROSCOPY

Bright-field microscopy is the method used with the ordinary light microscope and is by far the most common technique for the observation of cell anatomy. The study of tissue structure under the light microscope is termed histology.

In the light microscope, natural light or light from an electric lamp is focused on the specimen by the condenser lens. The illuminated image of the specimen is then enlarged, first by the objective lens and secondly by the projector lens (eyepiece) through which the observer sees the final magnified image (Fig. 1.1a).

For most general purposes, the ordinary light microscope provides adequate information about the structure of cells, and all the micrographs in subsequent chapters in this book have been obtained with this technique. Furthermore, numerous specific staining techniques (called cytochemical methods) exist for identifying, under the light microscope, certain chemical constituents in the cell. Thus, the distribution, for example, of carbohydrates, fats, proteins, nucleic acids and enzymes can now not only be accurately determined but also be quantified using microspectrophotometry (Pollister *et al.,* 1969; Pattison *et al.,* 1979). There are, however, two drawbacks in the use of ordinary light microscopy:

(1) Living cells cannot be studied in any detail.
(2) The resolution is limited.

1.2   PHASE-CONTRAST MICROSCOPY AND OTHER TECHNIQUES

Most living tissues are too thick to allow light to pass through them and form an image under the light micro-

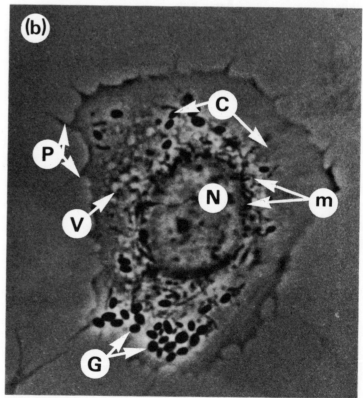

Fig. 1.2.   Two similar animal blood cells viewed under (a) bright-field and (b) phase optics, respectively. Nucleus (N), cytoplasm (C), granules (G), mitochondria (m), vacuoles (V) and pseudopodia (P). Micrograph (a) ×1800, (b) × 2300. *See* text for details. (Micrograph (b) courtesy of A. F. Rowley.)

scope. In consequence, animal tissues have to be processed, cut into sections and then stained (*see* Chapter 2) before their structure can be examined. Unfortunately, during these treatments, the tissue is killed, and the original structure may thus be altered and artefacts introduced into the specimen. Fortunately, a few mammalian tissues are sufficiently thin to allow the transmission of light so that they can be examined in the living state without prior treatment. A drop of blood, for example, can be diluted and placed directly onto a slide and examined. For such studies, the light microscope has been modified and special techniques such as phase-contrast microscopy have been introduced. In phase-contrast microscopy, a phase plate is introduced into the objective and an annulus is placed below the condenser of an ordinary light microscope. The overall effect of these modifications is to magnify the differential retardation of the light waves which occurs as they pass through the various components of the specimen (for further details, *see* Bradbury, 1976).

Figures 1.2a and 1.2b show the final images obtained of two similar animal cells viewed under bright-field and phase-contrast microscopy, respectively. In Fig. 1.2a the cell has been fixed in formaldehyde, stained with Giemsa stain (*see* section 2.1.7(i)) and photographed under bright-field optics. In Fig. 1.2b a similar cell has been examined in a fresh, living preparation and photographed under phase-contrast optics. It can be seen that under phase contrast it is generally much easier to make out details of the cell organelles than under ordinary light

microscopy, in which fixation precipitates and cross-links the cellular constituents and may obscure cellular detail. Furthermore, movements of the living cells and their constituents can also be studied under phase microscopy.

Phase-contrast microscopy is of special value in tissue culture experiments during which thin layers or suspensions of cells are maintained in nutrient media. Such cultured cells are regularly examined under phase-contrast microscopy in order to determine cell numbers, viability, movements, cellular interactions, etc.

Other, less commonly used, techniques for studying living cells, which were popular before the advent of the phase-contrast microscope, include vital staining methods for the staining of living cells and their examination under bright-field microscopy. Various interference and polarising microscopes (*see* Bradbury, 1976) have also been developed for examining living cells. Nomarski interference microscopy is particularly useful and gives a three-dimensional image (Fig. 1.3), while polarising microscopy can be employed to examine cellular components which are arranged in a highly ordered fashion, such as crystals and bundles of tubules or filaments.

1.2.1 Limits of resolution

Resolution in the light microscope is limited to $0.1–0.2\,\mu$m so that structural details of cell organelles cannot be obtained with this technique. The resolving power of a microscope is the amount of fine detail that can be

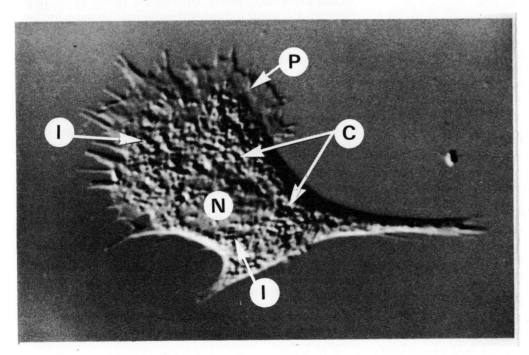

Fig. 1.3. Living animal blood cell photographed under Nomarski interference optics. Nucleus (N), cytoplasm (C), cytoplasmic inclusions (I) and pseudopodia (P). ×1900. (Courtesy of A. F. Rowley.)

discerned in a specimen. The higher the resolution, the more fine detail will be made out. Resolution in the light microscope is determined by the wavelength of the light source together with the numerical aperture of the objective lens and is represented by

$$\text{Resolution} = \frac{\text{Wavelength of light source} \times 0.6}{\text{Numerical aperture of objective lens}}$$

which is usually written as

$$r = \frac{0.6\lambda}{n\sin\alpha}$$

where r is the resolution, 0.6 is a constant, λ is the wavelength of the light source, and $n\sin\alpha$ is the numerical aperture of the objective lens.

The numerical aperture of an objective lens is a measure of the amount of light gathered by that lens. When the objective is close to the specimen (as in high-power objectives), more light will be gathered and resolution will be higher than when the objective is a long way from the specimen (as in low-power objectives).

From the above formula, the resolving power of the microscope can be calculated. The wavelength of visible light is about $0.5\,\mu$m and the numerical aperture of the best oil immersion lens is approximately 1.4, so that we have

$$r = \frac{0.6 \times 0.5}{1.4} = 0.2\,\mu\text{m.}$$

This figure of $0.2\,\mu$m is the best resolution that can be obtained with an expensive research microscope. In practice, the average class microscope, assuming that it is correctly aligned, will probably have a resolution of 0.4–$0.5\,\mu$m. However, if the thickness of the coverslip exceeds 0.17 mm and there is excessive mountant present (a common failing with inexperienced students), then the resolution will be reduced even further.

The term 'resolution' should not be confused nor used interchangeably with the term 'magnification'. The magnification of a specimen under any microscope simply represents the amount of enlargement, such as ×400, and this figure tells you absolutely nothing about the amount of detail visible. Most microscopes are capable of magnifying a specimen ×400 but there is no point in enlarging to this extent if the final image is blurred, which it will be if the resolving power of the objective lens has been exceeded.

The only way of improving the resolution of the microscope is to use an illumination source of shorter wavelength. The need for improved resolution thus led to the development of the electron microscope, during the late 1920s and early 1930s, in which an electron beam of extremely short wavelength is used to illuminate the specimen.

1.3　ELECTRON MICROSCOPY

Figure 1.1b shows that the layout of the electron microscope is basically similar to that of the light microscope. The electron gun takes the place of the electric lamp but both condenser and objective lenses are present, serving to focus the 'light' source and magnify the specimen, respectively. These lenses are not glass but are magnetic, and, since the eye is insensitive to electrons, the final image is not observed directly but is projected onto a fluorescent screen.

Another important difference between light and electron microscopes is that the latter always operate under vacuum because of the poor penetration power of electrons in air. This makes the electron microscope a cumbersome and expensive instrument and has for years prevented the study of living specimens (*see,* however, Parsons, 1974). A further disadvantage results from the limited penetration power of electrons, even in a vacuum, so that only very thin sections of specimens can be utilised. Sections must be as thin as 50–100 nm (0.05–0.1 μm), i.e. about 100 times thinner than the 5–10 μm wax sections cut for the light microscope. This necessitates the use of special embedding resins, such as the epoxy resins (e.g. Epon and Araldite), to provide adequate support for the specimen because wax can only be sectioned satisfactorily down to $1 - 2$ μm. Furthermore, the sections must be cut on expensive ultramicrotomes with glass or diamond knives.

In summary, the specialised nature of specimen processing for electron microscopy is time consuming and requires a high degree of skill to obtain satisfactory results (*see* Glauert, 1975, for a complete guide to the preparation of biological material for electron microscopy). The introduction of high-voltage electron microscopy (reviewed by Swann *et al.*, 1974) in recent years does mean that sections several micrometres thick can now be studied and, although, to date, resolution is rather poor, living material held in special chambers in the microscope column can be examined.

Assuming that the specimen preparation is optimal and taking into account the wavelength of the electron beam, which is of the order of 0.005 nm, then with biological specimens a resolution of 1–1.5 nm can be obtained in the electron microscope. This is 100–150 times greater than the optimal resolution in the light microscope. Furthermore, the electron microscope can magnify in excess

Fig. 1.4.(a)

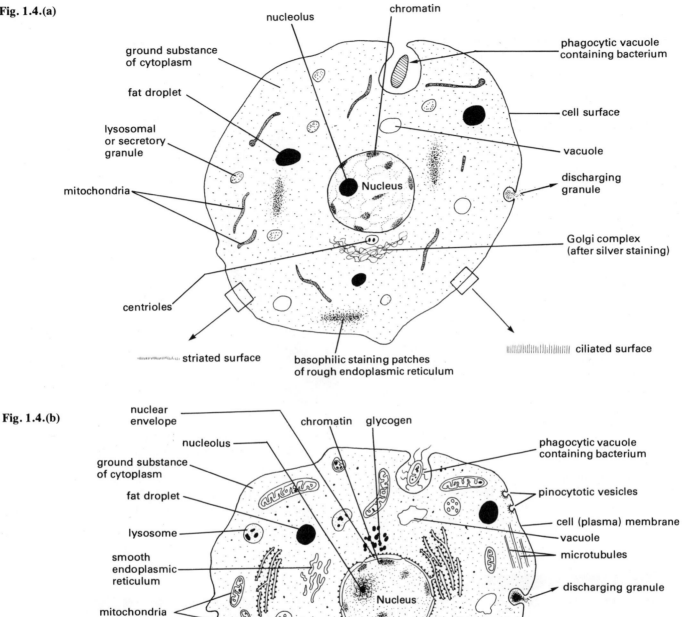

nucleolus

chromatin

phagocytic vacuole
containing bacterium

ground substance
of cytoplasm

cell surface

fat droplet

vacuole

lysosomal
or secretory
granule

discharging
granule

Nucleus

mitochondria

Golgi complex
(after silver staining)

centrioles

striated surface

basophilic staining patches
of rough endoplasmic reticulum

ciliated surface

Fig. 1.4.(b)

nuclear
envelope

chromatin

glycogen

nucleolus

phagocytic vacuole
containing bacterium

ground substance
of cytoplasm

pinocytotic vesicles

fat droplet

cell (plasma) membrane

lysosome

vacuole

smooth
endoplasmic
reticulum

microtubules

discharging granule

mitochondria

multivesicular
body

basal body of cilium

Nucleus

centrioles in
transverse and
longitudinal section

cilia

secretory
granule

Golgi complex

microvilli
(= striated border in (a))

free ribosomes

desmosome

rough endoplasmic reticulum

Fig. 1.4. Two generalised animal cells viewed (a) under light microscopy and (b) under electron microscopy. Note how much additional detail can be obtained of cell structure under the electron microscope

of 200000 times, although magnification of 40000–60000 times usually gives maximal resolution.

1.3.1   Fine structure of mammalian cells

Utilising the much-enhanced resolving power of the electron microscope, the fine structure of cells has been described. The following is a brief account of cell ultrastructure together with examples of electron micrographs of representative tissues found in the mammalian body. Complete reviews of mammalian cell ultrastructure can be found in many textbooks, including Rhodin (1963), Bloom and Fawcett (1968) and Novikoff and Holtzmann (1976).

Figure 1.4b illustrates the fine structure of a generalised animal cell and demonstrates quite clearly the additional information that can be obtained by using electron microscopy rather than light microscopy as in Fig. 1.4a.

The main cellular components observed under the electron microscope are the plasma membrane, the nucleus, the cytoplasmic organelles, which include the mitochondria, endoplasmic reticulum, Golgi complex, lysosomes, microtubules, microfilaments, lipid droplets, secretory granules, glycogen inclusions and centrioles, and specialisations of the cell periphery such as the microvilli, cilia and junctional complexes.

(a) Plasma membrane

The outer limiting membrane of the cell is the plasma membrane which serves to regulate the interaction of the cell with its environment. Similar membranes are found around many of the cellular components. The plasma membrane is *not* visible under the light microscope and the electron microscope has shown that it is about 7–10 nm thick and composed of three layers (Fig. 1.5).

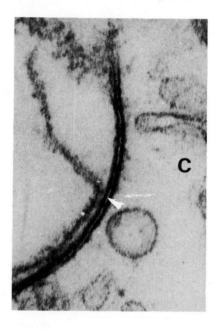

Fig. 1.5.
Structure of plasma membrane as seen under the electron microscope. Note transparent layer (arrow) sandwiched between two dense layers. Cytoplasm (C). ×225 000

The middle layer is transparent to electrons and is sandwiched between an outer and an inner electron-dense layer (Fig. 1.5). This apparently simple structure led earlier microscopists to hypothesise that the central layer was composed of a bilayer of lipid, covered on its inner and outer surfaces by a layer of protein (Fig. 1.6a). In such

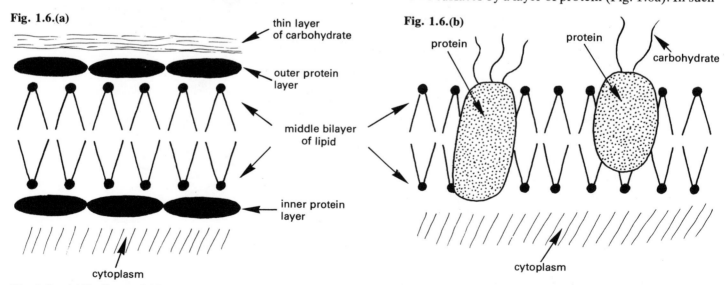

Fig. 1.6.(a)

thin layer of carbohydrate

outer protein layer

middle bilayer of lipid

inner protein layer

cytoplasm

Fig. 1.6.(b)

protein

protein

carbohydrate

cytoplasm

Fig. 1.6.   (a) Earlier model for the structure of the plasma membrane. (b) More recent model for structure of the plasma membrane

a model, the protein layers would be relatively immobile. However, more recent research has shown that the protein and glycoprotein (= protein plus attached carbohydrate) in the plasma membrane are in actual fact highly mobile and the so-called 'fluid mosaic' model for membrane structure was proposed (Fig. 1.6b) (Singer and Nicolson, 1972). In this model, the proteins are inserted into or 'float' at different depths in a lipid bilayer (Fig. 1.6b) and can thus rapidly move laterally over relatively long distances. Thus the receptors on the surfaces of cells, which are formed by the 'floating' proteins plus a carbohydrate component, can be shown, with appropriate markers, to aggregate rapidly following various treatments, e.g. exposure to metabolic poisons.

(b) The nucleus

The nucleus is bounded by two closely apposed membranes, the inner and outer nuclear membranes, which together form the nuclear envelope (Fig. 1.7). Each of these membranes has a similar ultrastructure to the outer plasma membrane of the cell, except that the outer nuclear membrane is often studded with ribosomes. At regular intervals, the nuclear envelope is perforated by pores (Fig. 1.7), which allow for the interchange of materials between the nucleus and the cytoplasm. Within the nucleus, often the most obvious feature is one or more large, electron-dense spherical accumulations of granules and fibrils called the nucleoli (Fig. 1.7). Each nucleolus is composed of both ribonucleic acid (RNA) and protein,

and is responsible for the synthesis of the RNA of the cytoplasmic ribosomes. Chromatin material is also present in the nucleus and forms numerous small particles and strands which in the interphase cell are scattered (= euchromatin) throughout the nucleoplasm or concentrated into small electron-dense clumps (heterochromatin) (Fig. 1.7). Chromatin is composed of protein and deoxyribonucleic acid (DNA) and represents the dispersed chromosomes which only during mitosis become condensed and clearly defined (Fig. 1.8). The protein subunits (= histones) are arranged into octomers around which are wrapped a length of DNA to form the nucleosomes. The nucleosomes thus appear as bead-like structures along the length of the chromatin and are interconnected by DNA.

(c) Mitochondria

Under phase-contrast optics of the light microscope, mitochondria appear as minute, structureless, filaments or rods (Fig. 1.2b), $1–5\,\mu$m long. The electron microscope, however, reveals their true complexity and shows that each mitochondrion is bounded by a double membrane separated by a space. The inner membrane is thrown into a number of folds, the cristae, which project into the inner compartment of the mitochondrion, the matrix (Fig. 1.9). The matrix also contains ribosomes, DNA fibrils and large electron-dense granules composed of divalent cations such as Ca . Mitochondria are the respiratory centres of the

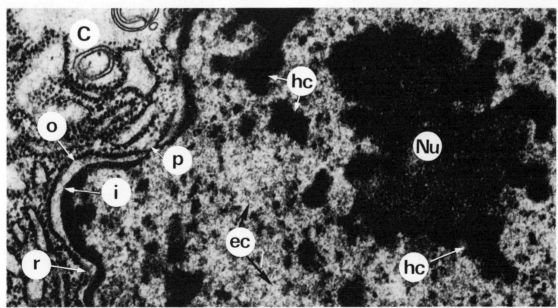

Fig. 1.7.   Nucleus of a digestive cell showing outer (o) and inner (i) nuclear membranes, a nucleolus (Nu), heterochromatin (hc) and euchromatin (ec). Note also the ribosomes (r) attached to the outer membrane and the presence of a nuclear pore (p) which is apparently closed by a thin membrane. Cytoplasm (C). ×59 000

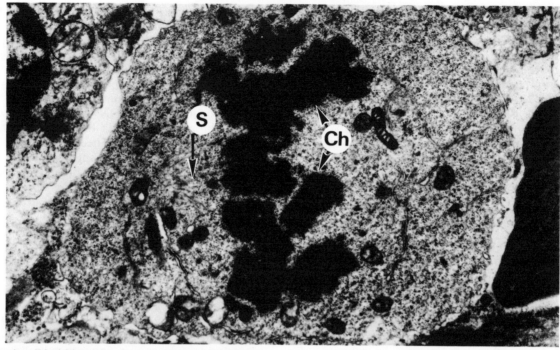

Fig. 1.8.   Mitotic cell in white pulp of spleen. Note condensed chromosomes (Ch) and microtubules of spindle (S). The nuclear envelope and nucleolus have disappeared at this stage. ×13 250

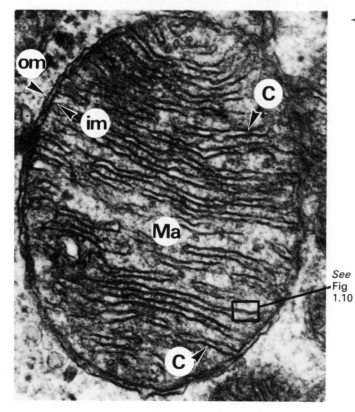

◄ **Fig. 1.9.**   Mitochondrion from rat diaphragm. The outer (om) and inner (im) mitochondrial membranes are separated by a narrow space. The inner membrane is infolded to form cristae (C) which project into the matrix (Ma). ×96 000

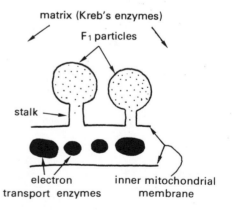

Fig. 1.10.   Diagram of portion of inner mitochondrial membrane such as that boxed in Fig. 1.9 showing distribution of respiratory enzymes following negative staining

cell and the various enzymes involved are located at different sites (Fig. 1.10). Many of the Krebs cycle enzymes are present in the matrix, while enzymes involved in phosphorylation and electron transport occur in the inner mitochondrial membrane. If mitochondria are exposed to osmotic shock, e.g. by negative staining, numerous small particles with stalks appear over the surface of the inner membrane (Fig. 1.10). These particles are called F_1 particles and are thought to contain an ATPase involved in ATP production (i.e. phosphorylation). The electron transport enzymes, however, remain embedded within the inner membrane (Fig. 1.10) and cannot be visualised.

(d) Endoplasmic reticulum and ribosomes

Many cells have an interconnecting network of membrane-delimited flattened sacs, tubules and vesicles called the endoplasmic reticulum. The endoplasmic reticulum is not usually visible in the light microscope, but in cells in which the network of membranes is well developed it may be detected by specific staining methods. Two types of endoplasmic reticulum exist and are often confluent:

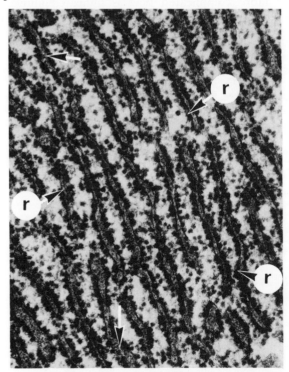

Fig. 1.11. Rough endoplasmic reticulum from rat pancreas cell. Numerous ribosomes (r) are attached to the outer surfaces of the membranes. Electron-dense secretory product (unlabelled arrows) is present in the lumen of the organelle. ×60 000. (Courtesy of A. F. Rowley.)

(1) Rough, or granular, endoplasmic reticulum (RER) in which the outer surfaces of the component membranes are studded with ribosomes (Fig. 1.11).
(2) Smooth, or agranular, endoplasmic reticulum (SER) which as its name implies is smooth and devoid of attached ribosomes (Fig. 1.12).

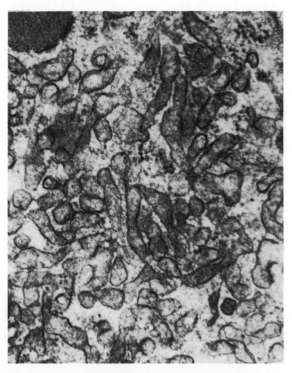

Fig. 1.12. Smooth endoplasmic reticulum from tracheal cell of rat. The component membranes are devoid of ribosomes. ×63 000

Since ribosomes are the sites of protein synthesis in the cell, then RER is particularly well developed in protein-secreting cells such as those of the pancreas (Figs. 1.11 and 1.25), and its general location in these cells can be detected under the light microscope with basic dyes (Fig. 1.4a). Ribosomes are usually bound to the membranes of the endoplasmic reticulum in cells in which the protein is synthesised for export. Each ribosome is composed of a large and a small subunit. The large subunit has many functions, including the binding of the ribosome to the membranes of the endoplasmic reticulum. It is also the site of peptide bond formation between amino acids, provides the energy for peptide formation and is responsible for movement of the polypeptide chain along the messenger RNA. The small subunit is the site of initiation of protein synthesis, of the interaction of messenger and transfer RNA and of the binding of transfer RNA. The newly synthesised polypeptide chain moves through a tunnel in the large ribosomal subunit and thence through another tunnel, composed of specific receptors, into the lumen of the endoplasmic reticulum. The endoplasmic reticulum then transports the protein to the Golgi complex for concentration, modification and packaging into secretory granules (Fig. 1.25). These granules pass to the cell periphery where they are discharged by exocytosis. In cells utilising large amounts of protein in growth processes, such as rapidly differentiating embryonic and tumour cells, numerous ribosomes are found free or associated in groups (= polyribosomes or polysomes) in the cytoplasm.

Smooth endoplasmic reticulum abounds in cells involved in lipid metabolism and is particularly common in steroid-hormone-producing cells such as those of the adrenal cortex. The SER is usually composed of small groups of membranous tubules rather than of flattened sacs of the sort characterising the RER (Figs 1.11 and 1.12).

(e) Golgi complex

The Golgi complex consists of stacks of smooth, membrane-bound, flattened sacs, and is usually present in the perinuclear region (Fig. 1.13). This organelle can be detected under the light microscope but only after staining with silver salts (Fig. 1.4a) or osmium tetroxide. Each Golgi body may contain several stacks of sacs and each stack often has a convex and a concave surface. The convex surface is usually unremarkable and is referred to as the immature face of the Golgi, while in the concave surface or mature face the margins of the component flattened sacs are frequently swollen, pinched off to form vesicles and vacuoles which eventually increase in electron density and give rise to secretory granules (Fig. 1.13). The Golgi complex is in intimate association with the RER from which membranous vesicles bud off, lose their ribosomes and fuse with the immature face of the Golgi. These 'transfer' vesicles serve to replace the Golgi membranes which are constantly being budded off at the mature face during the formation of the secretory granules. They also transfer the newly synthesised protein from the RER to the Golgi body for subsequent processing. The Golgi complex not only packages this protein into granules but also may add its own carbohydrate product to the secretion. The function of the Golgi body, however, is rather more complicated than is indicated above. For example, recently it has been shown that in some cells

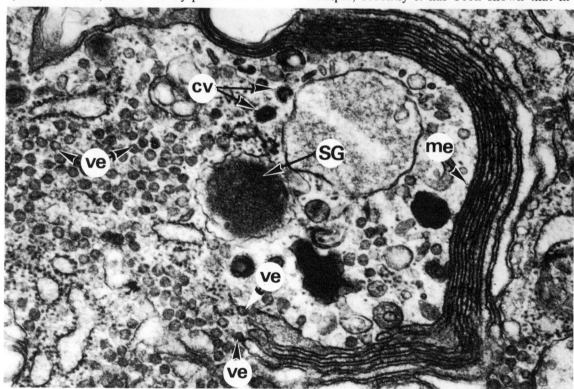

Fig. 1.13.   Golgi body from digestive cell. The membranes (me) at the margins of the concave surface are budding off numerous vesicles (ve) some of which eventually probably coalesce to form secretory granules (SG) of the sort indicated. Coated vesicles (cv). ×57 000

different types of secretory granules can be formed from the mature and immature faces of the same Golgi complex, so that these two regions of the same organelle must have a different enzyme component.

(f) Lysosomes

Lysosomes are a heterogeneous population of spherical, membrane-bound organelles, $0.25–5\,\mu\text{m}$ in diameter, which can be clearly seen under the light microscope (Fig. 1.4a). They contain one or more of a whole range of acid hydrolases but are characterised by the presence of acid phosphatase activity (Fig. 1.14). These enzymes

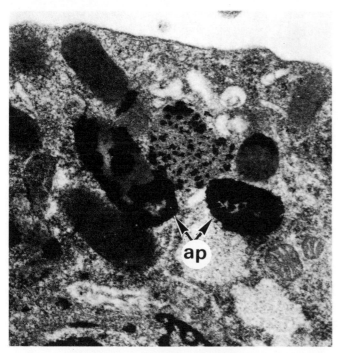

Fig. 1.14. Group of lysosomes from blood cell. They have been localised by their content of acid phosphatase (ap) which has bound a dense lead deposit here. ×49 000. (Courtesy of A. F. Rowley.)

reflect the function of lysosomes, which is intracellular digestion. The enzymes within lysosomes are synthesised by the Golgi complex and/or the Golgi-associated endoplasmic reticulum (GERL) and are budded off the Golgi as small vesicles called primary lysosomes. Foreign material, such as bacteria, is phagocytosed at the cell surface and comes to lie within a phagocytic vacuole or phagosome in the cytoplasm (Fig. 1.15). The primary lysosomes fuse with the phagosome and discharge their contents into the vacuole, thus forming a phagolysosome within which killing and digestion of the foreign body take place.

Breakdown of foreign materials may be incomplete and indigestible products may accumulate in the phagolysosome, which is now referred to as a residual body. Residual bodies are frequently highly pigmented and their contents may be discharged from the cell by exocytosis. Phagolysosomes can be labelled by feeding cells in culture with electron-opaque markers such as colloidal gold (Fig. 1.15).

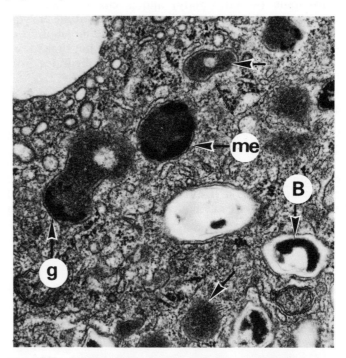

Fig. 1.15. Secondary lysosomes from mouse macrophage labelled with colloidal gold (g). Unlabelled lysosomes (unlabelled arrows) and phagocytosed bacteria (B) are also present in this cell. Note the membrane (me) around the lysosomes. ×40 000

Under certain conditions such as starvation, injury or ageing, portions of the cells' own cytoplasm may become enclosed within a membrane and degraded by the lysosomal enzymes. In this situation, the primary lysosomes fuse with a vacuole containing mitochondria, RER, etc., and form an autophagic vacuole, and again the indigestible remnants may accumulate to form residual bodies. Phagolysosomes, autophagic vacuoles and residual bodies are sometimes referred to collectively as secondary lysosomes.

White blood cells (e.g. macrophages and polymorphs), in particular, have large numbers of lysosomes which are all-important in the killing and breakdown of ingested micro-organisms during the defence reactions of the body to would-be invaders causing disease.

The products of lysosomal digestion can be re-utilised by the cell and, since they are usually of relatively low molecular weights, they can diffuse directly from the lysosomes into the surrounding cytoplasm.

In many cells of the body, and in the liver and kidneys in particular, another organelle is found which is about the same size as lysosomes, has a bounding membrane and contains various enzymes. This structure is called the peroxisome (= microbody) and is characterised by a central crystalline core and/or the presence of the enzyme catalase. Peroxisomes are involved in the metabolism of hydrogen peroxide, and probably also in the breakdown of purines and in the formation of carbohydrates from fats.

(g) Microtubules and microfilaments

Microtubules are proteinaceous cylinders about 25 nm in diameter which often appear to be randomly dispersed throughout the cytoplasm of many cells (Fig. 1.16). They were only discovered in 1963 with the introduction of glutaraldehyde as a fixative in electron microscopy and are not normally visible under the light microscope unless

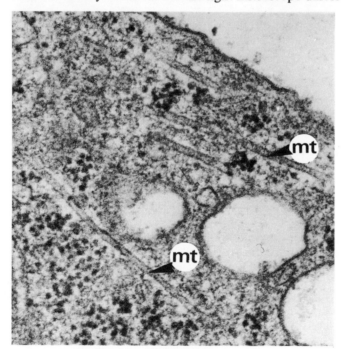

Fig. 1.16.   Microtubules (mt) in periphery of blood cell. ×88 000. (Courtesy of A. F. Rowley.)

they are associated in large bundles. Structurally, they are quite complex, with the wall of the cylinder formed by 13 protofilaments, composed of the proteins α- and β-tubulin, and arranged in a helical manner. Microtubules form a

cytoskeleton, control cell shape and are involved in cell movements. In some animal cells, microtubules serve to transport other organelles from one region of the cytoplasm to another. Thus, the transport of proteins and neurosecretory material from the cell body of neurones down the axons is probably effected by longitudinally oriented microtubules. Microtubules are also important components of centrioles, flagella and cilia (*see* below), and form the spindle during cell division.

Cells also contain microfilaments (Fig. 1.17) which are about 4–7 nm in diameter and composed of the fibrous protein, actin. Microfilaments are arranged in various

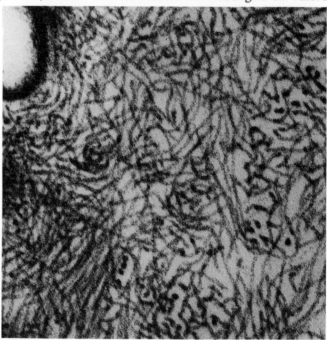

Fig. 1.17.   Microfilaments from a stratified epithelial cell of the ferret oesophagus. ×110 000

ways in different cell types but are particularly common in cells exhibiting cytoplasmic streaming and amoeboid movements. They often form parallel bundles in the cytoplasm, as in the tonofibrils of the skin, but frequently occur as complex webs beneath the plasma membrane. They also radiate out from the desmosomes which bind cells together (Fig. 1.24) and occur in the cores of the microvilli in the intestinal epithelium. Microfilaments have been shown to be involved in cytoplasmic streaming and by their contractions may actually propel the cytoplasmic matrix along. They also provide, like microtubules, a cytoskeletal system in the cell, and are involved in phagocytosis in which they may be essential for the formation of the small pseudopodia (= filopodia) to which foreign particles attach.

(h) Additional inclusions

Centrioles, glycogen and other secretory or storage products are commonly observed in cells. A pair of centrioles at right-angles to each other is often found in the cytoplasm adjacent to the nucleus. Each centriole is cylindrical with its wall composed of nine parallel groups of microtubules. There may be one, two or three micro-tubules in each group (Fig. 1.18). Just prior to cell division, the centrioles duplicate and each pair takes up a position at opposite poles of the nucleus. The nuclear membrane breaks down and the spindle, for attachment of the chromosomes, forms between the two pairs of cen-trioles (Fig. 1.8).

Cells also commonly contain secretory and/or storage products such as glycogen, lipid and zymogen granules. Glycogen is often particulate in form and may aggregate, as in the mammalian liver, to form rosettes (Fig. 1.19). Lipid (fat) droplets are stored in the cytoplasm of many cells and their appearance depends upon their degree of extraction by the solvents used in tissue processing for the electron microscope. When this dissolution is minimal, then the lipid appears as medium to electron-dense inclusions (Fig. 1.20), but if extraction is pronounced then

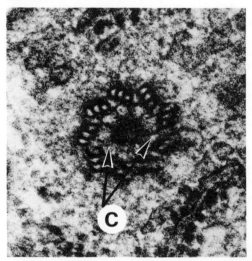

Fig. 1.18.   Transverse section of a centriole from a rat pancreatic cell. Note nine groups of microtubules, with each group containing three microtubules, forming the wall. A central cartwheel (C) is also just visible. ×130 000. (Courtesy of A. F. Rowley.)

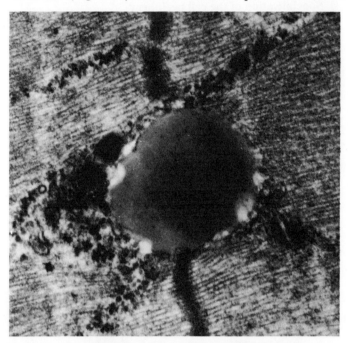

Fig. 1.20.   Lipid droplet in muscle of rat diaphragm. Note the lack of a bounding membrane. ×62 000

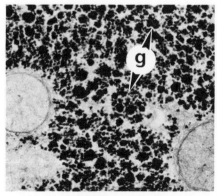

Fig. 1.19.   Glycogen rosettes (g) in mammalian liver cell. ×17 600. (Courtesy of J. G. Richards.)

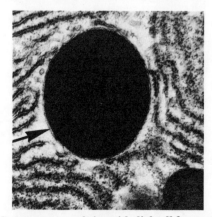

Fig. 1.21.   Secretory granule in epithelial cell from mouse trachea. Note outer limiting membrane (arrow). ×24 000

all that remains are electron-transparent spaces in the cytoplasm. Lipid droplets are not bound by a membrane and can thus be clearly distinguished from the membrane-bound secretory granules found in many cells (Fig. 1.21). For example, at the apices of the acinar cells of the pancreas, numerous secretory granules, called zymogen granules, are present which represent the precursors of the enzymes produced by this organ (Fig. 1.25).

(i) Specialisation of the cell periphery

Both the peripheral cytoplasm and the outer plasma membrane are frequently involved in .the formation of specialised organelles. These structures include the microvilli, cilia and junctional complexes, each of which serves a different purpose in the cell.

Microvilli, which are $0.5-1 \mu$m long, are delicate, finger-like extensions of the free surfaces of certain cells (Fig. 1.22). They form the striated surface (= brush border) of the intestinal epithelium, for example, and serve to increase the area for absorption. Sometimes, as in the ductus epididymis (Fig. 13.3), the microvilli are as long as cilia and, although they are non-motile, are referred to as stereocilia.

Cilia are motile cell extensions which are $5-10 \mu$m long and are found on the free surfaces of the epithelia lining, for example, the respiratory tract (Fig. 1.22), the fallopian tubes and the tympanic cavity. They serve to move substances, such as mucus in the trachea, across the surfaces of the cells, and to circulate fluids in confined spaces. Each cilium has an outer plasma membrane and is composed of nine pairs of longitudinally oriented microtubules, forming a ring around a pair of central tubules (Fig. 1.23). This is the so-called $9+2$ arrangement and, whereas the central pair of microtubules ends at the cell surface, the outer nine pairs extend into the peripheral cytoplasm and terminate in a modified centriole called the basal body. In the olfactory epithelium, the structure of the cilia is modified for sensory perception, and these organelles are extremely long (up to 200μm), are non-motile and have lost the usual $9+2$ arrangement of the microtubules.

Junctional complexes are localised modifications of the plasma membranes of adjacent epithelial cells and serve to anchor the cells together and to control the transepithelial movement of materials such as sugars and proteins through, for example, the endothelial cells lining the capillaries. Different types of junctional complexes exist, but one of the most commonly encountered forms is the desmosome (Fig. 1.24). Desmosomes (= macula adherens) are localised, disc-shaped areas of specialisation of the adjacent plasma membranes which appear more electron-dense than normal and from which a large number of microfilaments diverge into the surrounding cytoplasm (Fig. 1.24).

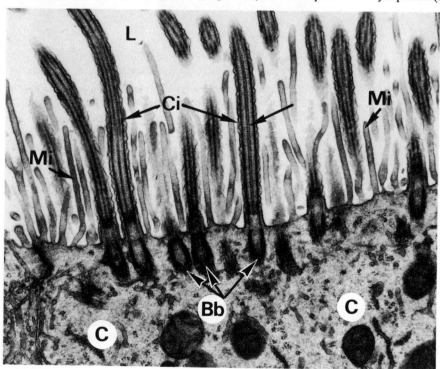

Fig. 1.22. Longitudinal sections of cilia (Ci) and microvilli (Mi) on the free surface of the columnar cells lining the trachea of a mouse. Note the basal bodies (Bb) and the central pair of microtubules (unlabelled arrow) of each cilium. Cytoplasm (C), and lumen of trachea (L). ×23 000

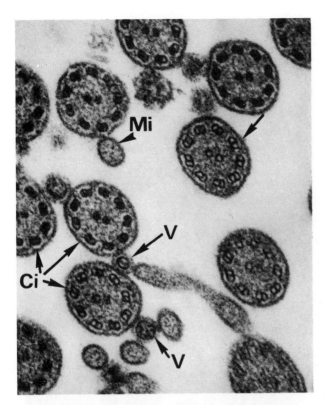

Fig. 1.23. Transverse sections through the cilia (Ci) and microvilli (Mi) of the columnar cells from the nasal mucosa of the ferret. The characteristic 9+2 arrangement of the microtubules in the cilia is clearly visible (unlabelled arrow). Note attached virus particles (V). × 90 000

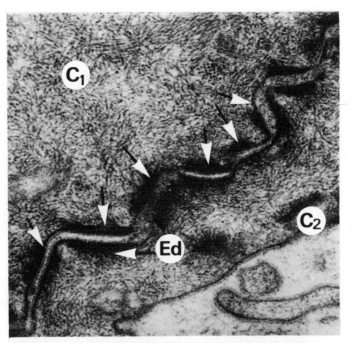

Fig. 1.24. A series of desmosomes (unlabelled arrows) is shown anchoring two adjacent cells (C₁ and C₂) from the ferret oesophagus. Note the increase in electron density (Ed) around each desmosome owing to large numbers of microfilaments diverging from these structures. × 76 000

1.4 ELECTRON MICROGRAPHS

In Figs 1.25 to 1.32 electron micrographs of representative tissues in the mammalian body are shown and clearly illustrate many of the organelles described above. Some of the electron micrographs are accompanied by light micrographs of thick plastic sections of the same tissue. Thick plastic sections are 0.5–2 μm sections of the same material that has been fixed and embedded in resin for thin sectioning for electron microscopy. Such thick plastic sections are stained and not only allow the orientation of embedded tissue to be determined prior to electron microscopy but also provide high-quality histological sections for light microscopy.

REFERENCES

Bloom, W. and Fawcett, D. W. (1968). *A Textbook of Histology,* 9th edn, W. B. Saunders, Philadelphia, London and Toronto.

Bradbury, S. (1976). *The Optical Microscope in Biology,* Institute of Biology's Studies in Biology, no. 59, Edward Arnold, London.

Glauert, A. M. (ed.) (1975). *Practical Methods in Electron Microscopy,* vol. 3, Elsevier/North-Holland Biomedical Press, Amsterdam.

Novikoff, A. B. and Holtzmann, E. (1976). *Cell and Organelles,* 2nd edn, Holt, Rinehart and Winston, New York.

Parsons, D. F. (1974). *Science,* **186**, 407–414.

Pattison, J. R., Bitensky, L. and Chayen, J. (eds) (1979). *Quantitative Cytochemistry and its Applications,* Academic Press, London.

Pollister, A. W., Swift, H. and Rasch, E. (1969). Microphotometry with visible light, in *Physical Techniques in Biological Research,* vol. 3C, ed. A. W. Pollister, Academic Press, New York and London, pp. 201–251.

Rhodin, J. A. G. (1963). *An Atlas of Ultrastructure,* W. B. Saunders, Philadelphia and London.

Singer, S. J. and Nicolson, G. L. (1972). *Science,* **175**, 720.

Swann, P. R., Humphreys, C. J. and Goringe, M. J. (eds) (1974). *Proc. 3rd Int. Conf. on High Voltage Electron Microscopy,* Academic Press, London.

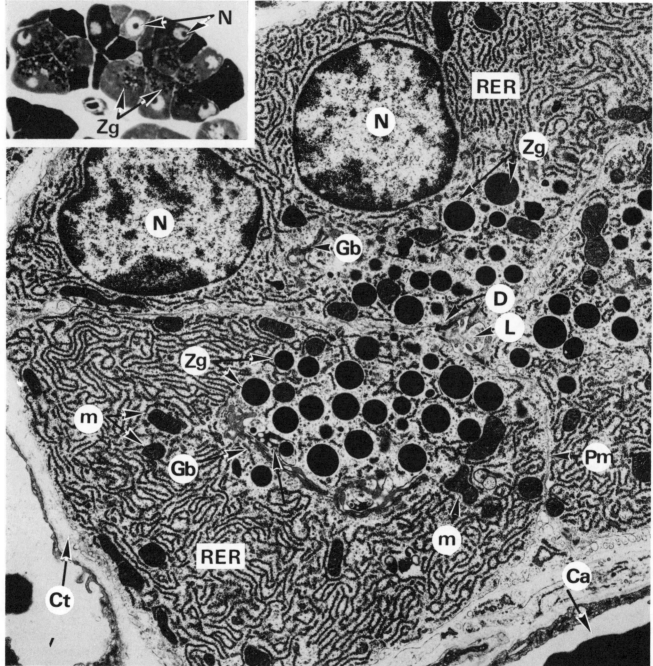

Fig. 1.25. Pancreas of rat. This electron micrograph shows the acinar cells which form the exocrine portion of the pancreas and are responsible for enzyme (i.e. protein) synthesis. Precursors of these enzymes are present at the apices of the cells in the form of zymogen granules (Zg) which discharge their contents into the central lumen (L). Other organelles present include an extensive rough endoplasmic reticulum (RER), prominent Golgi bodies (Gb) which can be seen packaging the secretory products of the RER into granules (unlabelled arrow). Mitochondria (m), desmosomes (D), adjacent plasma membranes (Pm), nuclei (N), connective tissue (Ct) and capillary (Ca). ×8000. (Courtesy of A. F. Rowley.) The inset shows, for comparative purposes, a thick plastic section. Zymogen granules (Zg) and the nuclei (N) are the most prominent features in these cells under the light microscope. ×800

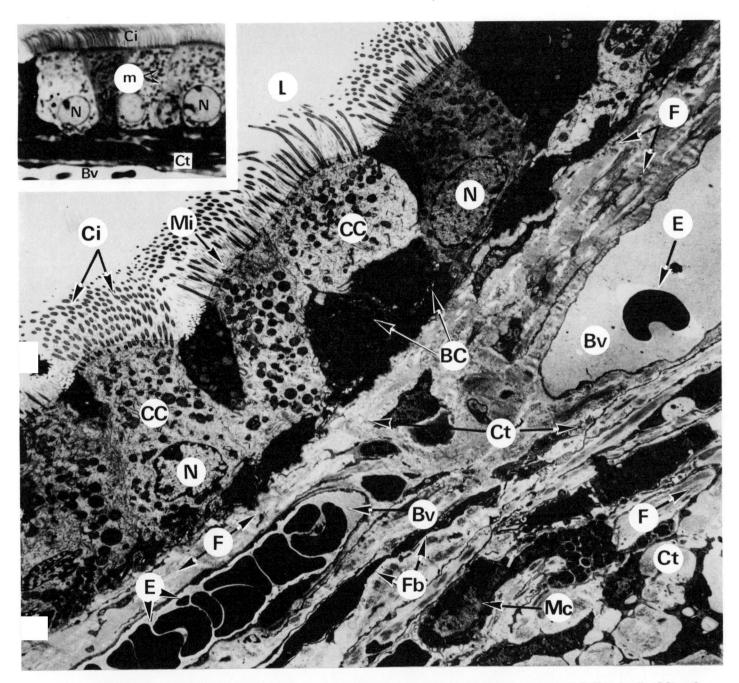

Fig. 1.26. Ciliated pseudostratified columnar epithelium of the mouse trachea. The epithelium is composed of ciliated cells (CC) and electron-dense basal cells (BC), and overlies a large amount of connective tissue (Ct) of the lamina propria which is composed of reticular and collagen fibres (F), fibroblasts (Fb), blood vessels (Bv) and a mast cell (Mc). Cilia (Ci), microvilli (Mi), lumen (L), nuclei (N) and erythrocytes (E). ×4000. The inset shows, for comparative purposes, a thick plastic section. Cilia (Ci), mitochondria (m), nuclei (N), connective tissue (Ct) and a blood vessel (Bv) are visible in this light micrograph. ×1300. (*N.B.* No goblet cells are shown in these micrographs.)

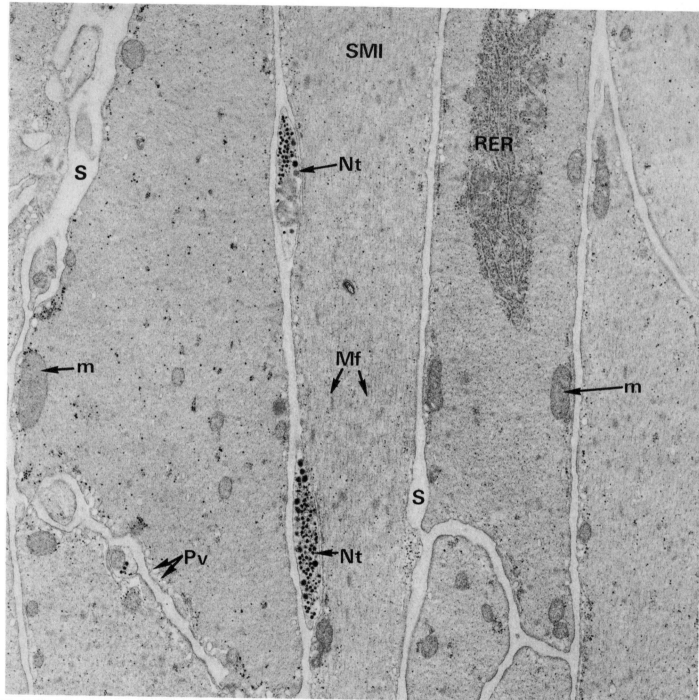

Fig. 1.27.   Smooth muscle cells from the vas deferens of the rat. The cells have been sectioned in different planes but the muscle cell at SMI is in longitudinal section and the cytoplasm (sarcoplasm) can be seen to be filled with parallel myofilaments (Mf). Mitochondria (m), rough endoplasmic reticulum (RER) and pinocytotic vesicles (Pv) are present. Note also that the cells are separated by a wide intercellular space (S) filled with amorphous material, and the adrenergic nerve terminals (Nt) containing synaptic vesicles which have been stained by the chromaffin reaction. ×21 600. (From *J. Histochem. Cytochem.*, 24, 1178-1193, by courtesy of J. P. Tranzer and J. G. Richards, and Elsevier/North-Holland Publ. Co.)

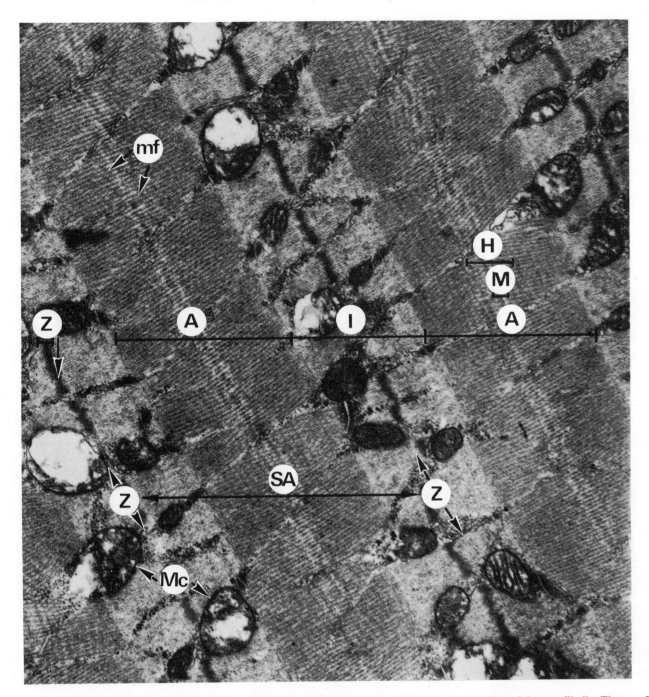

Fig. 1.28. Portion of striped muscle fibre from rat diaphragm showing the characteristic cross banding of the myofibrils. The myofibrils can be seen to be composed of fine microfilaments (mf). The extents of the M, H, A, I and Z bands are indicated, and the segment between two successive Z bands represents one sarcomere (SA). The H band is the lighter central region of an A band, while the M band is the narrow dark zone in the middle of the H band. Mitochondria (Mc). ×30 000

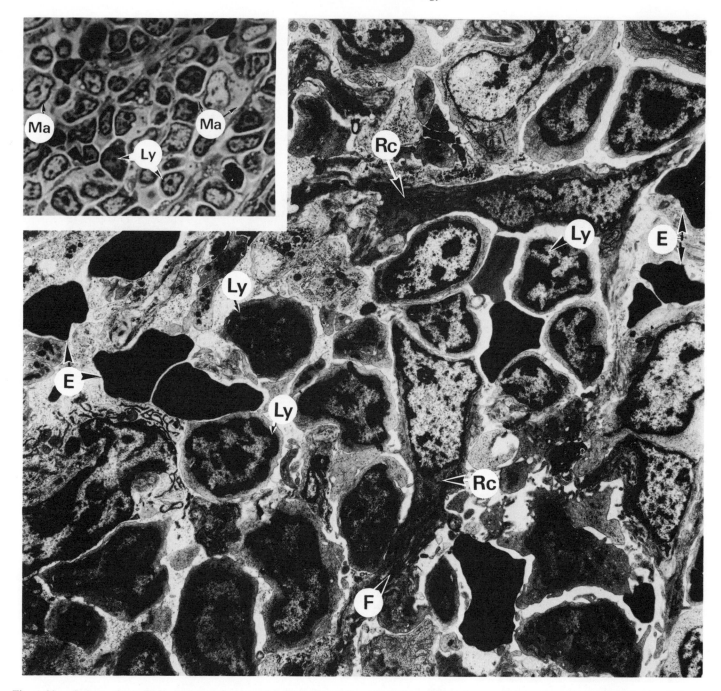

Fig. 1.29.   Spleen of rat. This electron micrograph is from the white pulp region of the spleen and shows numerous lymphocytes (Ly)
              interspersed with reticular cells (Rc) which produce reticular and collagen fibres (F). Erythrocytes (E). ×4500. The inset
              shows, for comparative purposes, a thick plastic section of a similar white pulp region. Lymphocytes (Ly) predominate in this
              light micrograph although larger cells which may represent fixed macrophage (Ma) are also present. ×1300

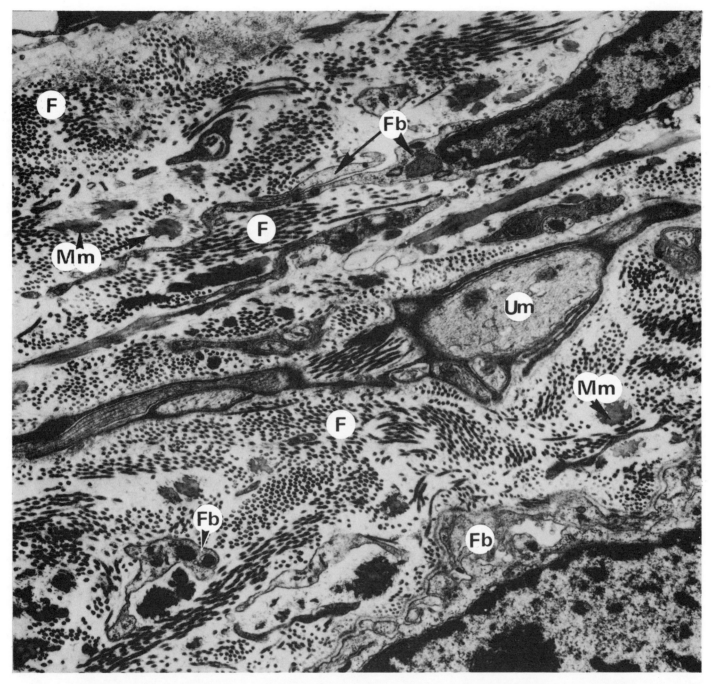

Fig. 1.30. Connective tissue and associated nervous tissue in the lamina propria of the mouse trachea. Note bundles of collagen fibres (F) sectioned in different planes, the fibroblasts (Fb) responsible for collagen production, amorphous matrix material (Mm) and the small unmyelinated nerve axon (Um). ×18 000

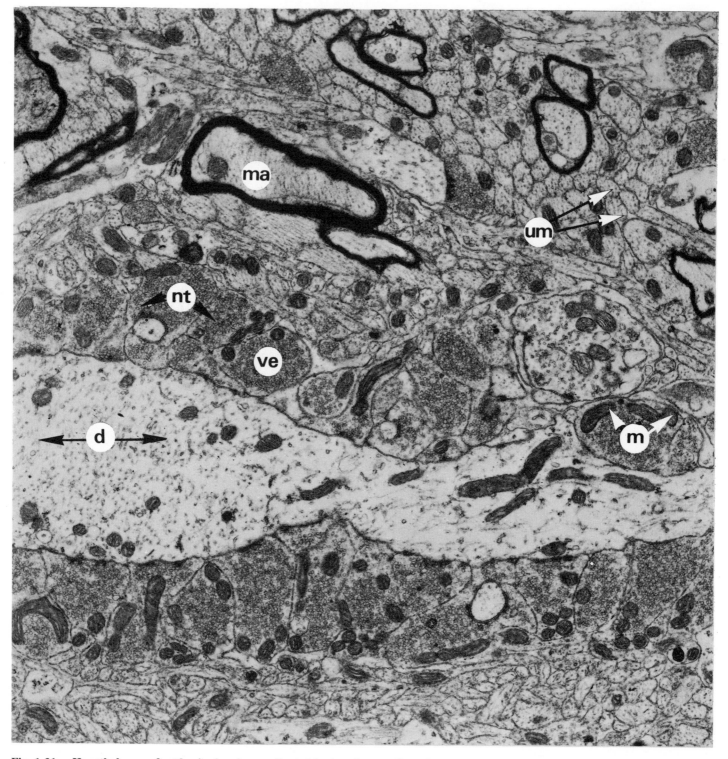

Fig. 1.31.   Hypothalamus of rat brain showing myelinated (ma) and unmyelinated (um) nerve axons, dendrite (d) and nerve terminals (nt) containing numerous vesicles (ve) and mitochondria (m). ×17 700. (Courtesy of J. G. Richards.)

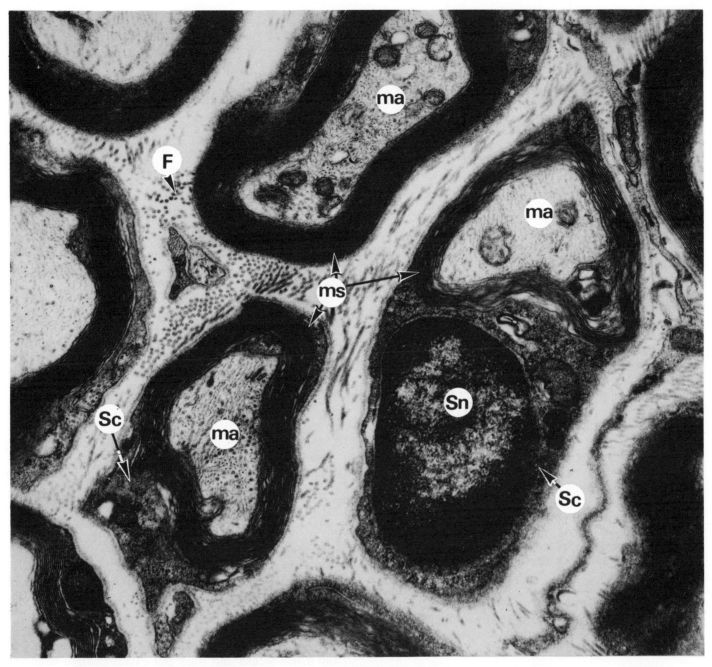

Fig. 1.32.   Myelinated nerve of mouse trachea. Note myelinated nerve axons (ma), myelin sheaths (ms) formed by the enveloping
Schwann cells (Sc), and the collagen fibres (F) of the endoneurium. Nucleus of Schwann cell (Sn). ×37 000

2 Some Useful Hints and Recipes for the Preparation and Examination of Stained Histological Sections

N.B. Many of the chemicals used in tissue processing are toxic

Since most mammalian organs and tissues cannot be examined *in situ* and are too thick to allow sufficient light to pass through them for microscopic examination, they must first be removed from the animal, cut into thin sections and then stained before their detailed structure can be examined under the compound light microscope. The following few pages contain a very brief outline of tissue preparation for the microscope and include some useful formulae and schedules which will hopefully assist the student in his laboratory work. Useful additional references for the more advanced student are also included.

2.1 TISSUE PROCESSING

The stages in the production of histological slides are:

(1) Fixation — preserves structure.
(2) Washing and dehydration — removes excess fixative and water which, if present, hinder later stages.
(3) Clearing — removes alcohol and allows wax infiltration.
(4) Wax infiltration and casting — supports tissue during sectioning.
(5) Section cutting (microtomy) and mounting.
(6) Staining — enhances contrast and introduces colour to specific regions of tissue.

2.1.1 Fixation

As soon as fresh tissues are removed from an animal, they begin to degenerate and break down because of the release of enzymes from the tissues themselves (autolysis) and also due to the activity of any contaminating bacteria. The tissue therefore soon loses its normal characteristic structure. In order to prevent such post-mortem changes, tissues are immersed in chemicals which inactivate the autolytic enzymes and kill the bacteria. Such chemicals, called fixatives, also assist in maintaining cellular structure by stabilising the constituents and rendering them insoluble in water and alcohol, to which the tissue is exposed during processing.

Many different chemical fixatives exist and usually act by cross-linking the proteins in the cells to preserve the *in vivo* (in life) structure. There are no perfect fixatives and many only preserve specific components such as the cytoplasm or the nucleus. Some very common fixatives are given below and most of the tissues in this book have been prepared using one or more of these.

(a) Formol saline

Sodium chloride	8.5 g
Formalin (40% aqueous)	100 ml
Distilled water	900 ml

Notes Use at pH 7.5–8.0; good general fixative but poor for testis; fix for 12–48 h and wash in several changes of 70% alcohol; tends to harden tissue.

(b) Bouin's fluid

Picric acid (saturated aqueous solution)	75 ml
Formalin (40% aqueous)	25 ml
Acetic acid (glacial)	5 ml

Notes Good general fixative but poor for kidney; cytoplasmic inclusions may be lost; fix for between 12 h and a few weeks and wash out excess fixative in several changes of 70% alcohol over 24 h. Sections can also be treated for 2–5 min in 70% alcohol saturated with lithium carbonate to remove excess fixative.

(c) Zenker's fluid

Mercuric chloride	5 g
Potassium dichromate	2.5 g

Sodium sulphate	1 g
Distilled water	100 ml
Glacial acetic acid	5 ml
(added just before use)	

Notes Good general fixative especially for cytoplasm; fix for 3–24 h and wash overnight in running tap water; then, to remove excess mercuric chloride from tissues, place for 5–6 h in 70% alcohol made dark brown by addition of saturated solution of iodine in 70% alcohol. If mercuric chloride crystals are still present in final stained sections, then, before staining, sections should also be immersed in Weigert's Lugol solution as follows:

Weigert's Lugol solution

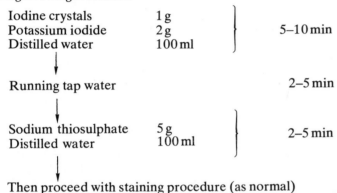

Iodine crystals	1 g		
Potassium iodide	2 g	}	5–10 min
Distilled water	100 ml		

| Running tap water | | 2–5 min |

| Sodium thiosulphate | 5 g | } | 2–5 min |
| Distilled water | 100 ml | | |

Then proceed with staining procedure (as normal)

(d) Hints for good fixation

(1) Select the fixative carefully. Although general fixatives exist (e.g. those in (a), (b) and (c) above), special fixatives for specific cell constituents, e.g. glycogen, nucleic acids, enzymes, etc., can be used.
(2) Place tissue in fixative *immediately* after removal from the animal.
(3) Generally, for good fixation, the tissue should be no thicker than approximately 0.5 cm. Larger pieces can be cut up in the fixative using sharp razors or scalpels. Large pieces of soft tissues, e.g. lung, liver, etc., will harden after 15–30 min in fixative and can then be cut down to the correct size.
(4) Use a volume of fixative at least 10–15 times the volume of the tissue.
(5) Use freshly made up fixatives.
(6) Make sure all fixative is *thoroughly* washed out before subsequent stages.

(e) Decalcification

The reader is referred to Wallington (1972). Bone and other calcified tissues cannot be satisfactorily sectioned unless the calcium salts are first removed. Many decalcifi-

cation methods exist, but usually acid or chelating agents are used *after fixation,* for example as follows:

Kristensen fluid

Formic acid (sp.gr. 1.2)	18 ml
Sodium formate	3.5 g
Distilled water	82 ml

Notes Fix, decalcify 24 h (spongy bone), or 5–10 days (compact bone); transfer directly to 70% alcohol, since prior washing in water is not required.

EDTA method

| Ethylene diamine tetra-acetic acid | 10 g |
| Distilled water | 90 ml |

Notes Neutralise above solution with sodium hydroxide pellets, fix, decalcify for 1–6 weeks, renew fluid every week, wash in 70% alcohol and process as normal.

Comment The chelating agent (EDTA) gives good staining after treatment but is very slow.

2.1.2 Washing and dehydration

Excess fixative must be removed or it will interfere with later stages. This can be accomplished, as indicated above, usually in running tap water or 50% or 70% alcohol, as appropriate.

Excess water must then be removed to allow subsequent infiltration of the tissue with molten wax. Water does not mix with wax and so would hinder the infiltration process. Dehydration is usually carried out in a graded series of ethanol, placing the tissue in 30%, 50%, 70%, 90% and absolute alcohol. The time in each varies according to the size of the tissue, but 1–2 h in each should be sufficient, pausing longer in absolute alcohol and making two or three changes over 2–3 h.

(a) Hints for dehydration

(1) Make sure the absolute alcohol does not contain excess water by mixing a few drops with xylene, which should remain clear; persistent cloudiness of xylene indicates excessive water present in the alcohol.
(2) Do not leave tissue in alcohol for too long, as extraction, and also hardening (making sectioning difficult), will occur.
(3) For dehydration, use industrial methylated spirit (74° O.P. grade = 95% ethanol) instead of absolute ethanol, which is expensive.

2.1.3 Clearing

Since alcohol does not mix with wax, it must be removed to allow wax infiltration. This is done by placing the tissue in a chemical that is miscible with molten wax, e.g. xylene, chloroform, cedarwood oil, etc. In xylene, 2–6 h is long enough, while cedarwood oil may take overnight or even longer. The tissue should become transparent. Milkiness indicates that water is still present, and that dehydration is unsatisfactory and should continue longer, perhaps with renewed absolute alcohol.

2.1.4 Wax infiltration and casting

In order to prevent the collapse and distortion of the tissue during sectioning, it must be impregnated and surrounded by hard wax for support. A simple infiltration procedure is the xylene method:

(1) From absolute alcohol → xylene (1 change)   2–6 h
(2) 50:50 xylene: wax — in oven (1 change)   1 h
(3) Molten wax* — in oven (3 changes)   1 h each

The tissue is now ready for casting into a solid block of wax which can be trimmed and fitted on a microtome. A convenient rapid way of embedding for small tissue blocks is the solid watchglass method. A deep solid watchglass is first smeared with glycerine and then filled with fresh molten wax. The wax in the centre is kept molten with a hot needle and the specimen transferred from the last wax change with *warm* forceps and oriented into the required position. The surface of the wax is solidified by gently blowing on it. When a thick skin has formed, the watchglass is slid at an angle into cold water (not iced). This will hasten solidification of the wax block, which can be removed from the water after 30 min and trimmed for microtomy. Many different sorts of paper or plastic containers can also be made or purchased for wax casting, especially for larger blocks of tissues.

(a) Hints for good wax embedding

(1) Make sure that fresh wax is used for casting the block and that it is at the correct temperature; semi-solid wax is most unsatisfactory.
(2) Do not overheat the wax, as this will harden the tissue before sectioning.
(3) Do not cool the block too quickly, as this will entrap air bubbles around the specimen.
(4) Always label the block with a slip of paper pushed into the edge of the molten wax.

(5) Difficult specimens, e.g. eyes, may require a special double embedding technique (*see* Humason, 1972).

2.1.5 Section cutting (microtomy) and mounting

The embedded tissue is trimmed into the form of a truncated pyramid, fixed to a specimen holder (this may just be a small cube of wood) which fits on the microtome, and sectioned with a sharp knife at approximately 6–8 μm. Details of microtomy are beyond the scope of this book (*see* Steedman, 1960) and can only be learned by adequate demonstration and practice.

(a) Hints for avoiding problems in microtomy

(1) To avoid curved ribbons of sections, make sure that the two horizontal edges of the block face are parallel to each other and also to the knife edge.
(2) Have a sharp knife at the correct angle for cutting.
(3) Do not cut in a draughty or very warm room.
(4) Always remove the knife from the microtome after use.
(5) Use a moist paint-brush to handle the sections.

Sections (2–3 per slide) are mounted on glass slides flooded with dilute albumen solution (= few drops egg albumen in 10–20 ml distilled water). Slides are then placed on a hotplate at about 50°C to allow sections to flatten, excess albumen solution is removed, and then the slides are dried overnight in an oven at approximately 30°C. Alternatively, sections can be flattened by placing on the surface of a water bath at 45–50°C and then picked up by passing a slide (coated thinly with undiluted albumen) under them and lifting it gently out of the water. Excess water is drained off *carefully* to avoid damaging the sections.

(b) Hints for avoiding problems in section mounting

(1) Place the ribbon of sections on the surface of a flat, fairly rough, preferably dark-coloured piece of paper after cutting.
(2) Make sure that the temperature of the surface of the hotplate is not higher than the melting point of wax.
(3) Always label your slides, preferably by means of a diamond marker, on the same surface as the sections are mounted.

Summary Schedule for Processing up to Staining

(1) Fix, e.g. formol saline, Bouin's or Zenker's, for 12–24 h.

---

* Different waxes are available but 'Fibrowax' (Raymond A. Lamb, London) is excellent and has a melting point of 57-58°C. Use of a vacuum oven during infiltration will assist penetration of wax into difficult tissues, e.g. skin, lung, etc.

(2) Wash in several changes of 70% ethanol for 6–24 h (formol saline and Bouin's) or in running tap water overnight (Zenker's).

(3) 70% ethanol for 1–2 h (+ saturated iodine for 5–6 h for Zenker's fixed material to remove mercuric chloride, then fresh 70% ethanol).

(4) 90% ethanol for 1–2 h.

(5) Absolute ethanol — several changes over 2–3 h.

(6) Xylene for 2–6 h.

(7) Xylene:wax (50:50) (in oven) for 1 h.

(8) Molten wax (in oven) — three changes, 1 h each.

(9) Embed in fresh wax.

(10) Trim block, mount on microtome, section at 6–8 μm.

(11) Flatten sections and mount *two* or *three* (only) on slides + adhesive, label slides.

(12) Dry slides overnight at approximately 30°C.

2.1.6 Staining — general method

The purpose of staining is to increase contrast between the various tissue and cell components. A whole range of different staining techniques is available, but the most widely used method is the *haematoxylin and eosin procedure*. Many of the tissues in this book have been stained by this method, which stains the nuclei dark blue with haematoxylin and the cytoplasm pink with the counterstain, eosin.

(a) Haematoxylin and eosin technique

Stains: nuclei — dark blue; and cytoplasm — pink.

(1)	Place slide in xylene to dewax	5–10 min
(2)	Absolute ethanol	2 min
(3)	90% ethanol	1 min
(4)*	70% ethanol	1 min
(5)	Ehrlich's haematoxylin (to stain nuclei *only*)	10–15 min
(6)	Blue in alkaline tap water (= weak bicarbonate solution)	5–10 min

(7) Examine (×5 or ×10 objective of microscope, wipe underside of slide and *do not* allow it to dry up)

    overstained (nuclei + cytoplasm also stained): remove excess stain in acid alcohol (2–3 s) and repeat steps (6) and (7)
    understained: replace in haematoxylin and repeat steps (6) and (7)

(8)	70% ethanol	2 min
(9)	Counterstain in 0.05% alcoholic eosin	3–6 min
(10)	Dip in 70% ethanol	few seconds

(11) Examine as in (7) above (wipe underside of slide and do not allow it to dry up)

    overstained (all section bright red and haematoxylin in nuclei masked):
      remove excess stain in 70% ethanol   2–3 s
    understained (cytoplasm very light pink):
      replace in eosin   2–3 min

(12)	90% ethanol	10–15 s
(13)	Absolute ethanol	2–3 min
(14)	Absolute ethanol	2–3 min
(15)	Clear in xylene (not the one used for dewaxing!)	5 min

(16) Mount in *one drop* Ralmount or D.P.X. (Raymond A. Lamb, London), do not allow slide to dry up at any stage.

Ehrlich's haematoxylin

Solution A

Haematoxylin	2 g	Dissolve haematoxylin
Absolute alcohol	100 ml	in alcohol

Solution B

Glycerine	100 ml	
Distilled water	100 ml	Dissolve
Aluminium potassium sulphate	in excess (approx. 20 g)	

Mix A and B together and add 10 ml glacial acetic acid. Ripens in approximately 8 weeks, when it turns dark red. Keeps for years.

Acid alcohol

70% ethanol	100 ml
Conc. hydrochloric acid	0.5 ml

Eosin counterstain
(Humason, 1972)

Eosin Y (C.I. No. 45380)	1 g
70% ethanol	1000 ml
Glacial acetic acid	5 ml

Dilute with equal volume of 70% ethanol and add 2–3 drops of glacial acetic acid. Keeps well.

Note Many other haematoxylins exist besides Ehrlich's, e.g. Harris's, Cole's, etc., and any of these may be used. Likewise, many workers prefer 1% aqueous eosin instead of the alcoholic eosin.

---

* If fixed in Zenker's, remove mercuric chloride in Lugol's solution (*see* section 2.1.1(c)), then proceed to (5).

(b)   Hints for haematoxylin and eosin staining

(1) Run a test slide through to determine optimal staining times, as these vary greatly depending upon fixative and tissue used, and age of stain.

(2) Mark side of slide on which section is mounted with diamond marker — this will prevent section being wiped off slide during examination for staining and wrong side of slide being mounted in (16).

(3) Before examining slide at (7) and (11) to determine staining, make *absolutely certain* that condenser of microscope is in correct position and that the iris diaphragm of the condenser is *fully open*.

(4) If section looks dark and 'watery' during (7) and (11), then either the microscope condenser is incorrectly positioned, the diaphragm is not fully open, or the slide has dried up.

2.1.7   Staining — specific methods used in this book and for the more ambitious student

Sometimes it may be necessary to use specific staining techniques in order to distinguish more clearly the different components of a tissue which unfortunately may stain very similarly with the haematoxylin and eosin technique. For example, connective tissue in organs such as the ovary and gut can be stained specifically with *Masson's trichrome method* and the various layers in these organs can then be more readily seen (e.g. *see* Fig. 14.1).

(a)   Masson's trichrome or triple method (Modified from Humason, 1972.)

For connective tissue in ovary or gut, for example. Stains three tissue components; nuclei—black; connective tissue—green; and cytoplasm—pink/red.

(1)	Place slide in xylene to dewax	5–10 min
(2)	Absolute ethanol	2 min
(3)	90% ethanol	1 min
(4)	70% ethanol	1 min
(5)	Hansen's iron trioxyhaematin	5–7 min
(6)	Examine (low power)	
	overstained: differentiate in acid alcohol (avoid overstaining if possible)	
	understained: replace in Hansen's	
(7)	Wash in running tap water	10–15 min
(8)	Acid fuchsin	5 min
(9)	Rinse in distilled water until excess stain removed	

(10)	Xylidine Ponceau (red) (overstaining slightly)	1–5 min
(11)	Differentiate in phosphomolybdic acid	5 min
(12)	Fast green (slightly overstaining connective tissue)	3 min
(13)	Rinse in distilled water until only connective tissue is green, leaving epithelium, muscle, etc., pink	
(14)	Rapid dehydration up ethanol series	0.5–1 s each
(15)	Absolute ethanol	3 min
(16)	Absolute ethanol	3 min
(17)	Clear in xylene (do not allow slide to dry up before mounting)	5 min
(18)	Mount in one drop Ralmount or D.P.X.	

Hansen's iron trioxyhaematin

Solution A

Iron alum (ammonium ferric sulphate)	10 g
Ammonium sulphate	1.4 g
Distilled water	150 ml

Solution B

Haematoxylin	1.6 g
Distilled water	75 ml

Dissolve solutions A and B by gentle heating. Add A to B (not vice versa), stirring constantly. Heat mixture slowly (without stirring) to boiling point. Cool rapidly. Original deep violet colour turns dark brown. If it has a green sheen, throw away. Filter and store in stoppered bottle with little air. Stores 6–8 months.

Acid fuchsin

Acid fuchsin	1 g
Glacial acetic acid	1 ml
Distilled water	100 ml

Xylidine Ponceau

Ponceau de xylidene	0.25 g
Glacial acetic acid	1 ml
Distilled water	100 ml

Phosphomolybdic acid

1% in distilled water

Fast green

Fast green	2 g
Glacial acetic acid	2 ml
Distilled water	100 ml

(b) Heidenhain's iron haematoxylin technique (After Smith and Bruton, 1978.)

For striations in muscle (*see* Fig. 6.1). Stains: nuclei — blue/black; and muscle striations — blue/grey.

(1) Dewax sections, bring sections to water and remove mercuric chloride (*see* haematoxylin and eosin technique in section 2.1.6(a)) if necessary
(2) Iron alum solution   0.5–24 h
(3) Rinse in tap water
(4) Stain in haematoxylin until section overall black (same length of time as in (2))   0.5–24 h
(5) Rinse in tap water
(6) Destain in iron alum solution (until nuclei and striations stand out), follow under microscope   1–30 min
(7) Wash in running tap water   10 min
(8) Dehydrate (70%, 90%, absolute ethanol), clear and mount

Iron alum

     5% ammonium ferric sulphate in distilled water

Haematoxylin

Haematoxylin	10 g
95% ethanol	100 ml

Stand until deep red colour (4–5 months). Add 5 ml of this stock to 100 ml distilled water before use.

(c) Heidenhain's azan technique (From Pantin, 1964.)

For differentiating between cell types in pituitary and pancreas, and cell layers in adrenals (*see* Figs 15.2 and 15.4). Stains: nuclei — red; collagen — blue; basophils — light blue; acidophils — orange/red; and chromophobes — colourless.

(1) Dewax sections, bring to water and remove mercuric chloride (*see* haematoxylin and eosin technique, section 2.1.6(a)) if necessary
(2) Stain in azocarmine at 56°C   1 h
(3) Wash in distilled water -   few seconds
(4) Differentiate in aniline alcohol under microscope — only nuclei pink/red
(5) Stop differentiation in acetic alcohol   0.5–1 min
(6) 5% phosphotungstic acid   1–3 h
(7) Wash *briefly* in distilled water

(8) Stain in Aniline Blue–Orange G   1–3 h
(9) Wash *briefly* in distilled water
(10) Differentiate in 96% ethanol
(11) Absolute ethanol, xylene and mount

Azocarmine

Azocarmine G	0.1 g
Glacial acetic acid	1 ml
Distilled water	100 ml

Boil azocarmine in distilled water; when cold, filter and add acetic acid.

Aniline alcohol

Aniline	1 ml
90% ethanol	1000 ml

Acetic alcohol

Glacial acetic acid	1 ml
90–95% ethanol	100 ml

Phosphotungstic acid

Phosphotungstic acid	5 g
Distilled water	100 ml

Make up fresh each time.

Aniline Blue–Orange G

Aniline Blue WS	0.5 g
Orange G	2.0 g
Distilled water	100 ml
Glacial acetic acid	8 ml

Add acetic acid last, boil, filter when cold and dilute with twice the volume of distilled water.

(d) Chromium–haematoxylin–phloxine technique (From Humason, 1972, after Gomori, 1941.)

For differentiating between different cell types in islets of Langerhans (*see* Fig. 11.20). Stains: beta cells — blue; alpha cells — red; delta cells — if present, red, like alphas.

(1) Tissue should initially be fixed in Bouin's; dewax sections and bring to water
(2) Refix in Bouin's   12–24 h
(3) Wash in running tap water   5 min
(4) Potassium dichromate–sulphuric acid   5 min
(5) Remove colour in 5% aqueous sodium bisulphite   3–5 min

(6)　Wash in running tap water　　　　　　5 min
(7)　Stain in haematoxylin until beta cells
deep blue　　　　　　　　　　　　　　10–15 min
(8)　Differentiate in 1% hydrochloric acid
(1 ml conc. HCl in 99 ml distilled water)　1 min
(9)　Wash in running tap water until clear
blue　　　　　　　　　　　　　　　　　5 min
(10)　Stain in phloxine　　　　　　　　　　5 min
(11)　Rinse briefly in distilled water
(12)　5% phosphotungstic acid (aqueous)　1 min
(13)　Wash in running tap water — sections
turn red　　　　　　　　　　　　　　　5 min
(14)　Differentiate in 95% ethanol. If
sections too red and blue alpha cells
not clear, rinse in 80% ethanol　　　　　15–20 s
(15)　Dehydrate, clear and mount

Potassium dichromate–sulphuric acid

Potassium dichromate	0.15 g
Distilled water	100 ml
Sulphuric acid (conc.)	0.5 ml

Phloxine

Phloxine B	0.5 g
Distilled water	100 ml

Haematoxylin solution

Haematoxylin	0.5 g
Distilled water	50 ml

When dissolved, add 50 ml of 3% aqueous potassium chromium sulphate. Mix well, then add:

Potassium dichromate (5% aqueous)	2 ml
0.5N sulphuric acid	2 ml

Allow to ripen 48 h, store at 4°C, filter before use.

(e)　Phloxine–tartrazine technique (From Smith and Bruton, 1978.)

For demonstrating Paneth cell granules in intestine (*see* Fig. 11.13). Stains: Paneth cell granules — bright red; nuclei — brown; and rest of tissues — yellow.

(1)　Dewax sections and bring to water
(2)　Stain in Mayer's haemalum　　　　　8 min
(3)　Blue in alkaline tap water (weak
bicarbonate solution)
(4)　Stain in phloxine　　　　　　　　　30 min
(5)　Rinse in water and blot *almost* dry

(6)　Counterstain in tartrazine (examine
under microscope)　　　　　　　　　　5–15 min
(7)　Rinse in water
(8)　Dehydrate in absolute ethanol, clear
and mount

Mayer's haemalum

Haematoxylin	1 g	Dissolve in distilled water with gentle heating
Sodium iodate	0.2 g	
Potassium alum	50 g	
Distilled water	1000 ml	

Shake frequently until solution is blue/violet (several hours). Then add:

Chloral hydrate	50 g
Citric acid	1 g

Solution should turn red/violet. Store in glass-stoppered bottle and leave at least 1–2 weeks before use.

Phloxine

Phloxine B	0.5 g
Calcium chloride (anhydrous)	0.5 g
Distilled water	100 ml

Tartrazine

Saturated solution of tartrazine in Cellosolve

(f)　Cajal method B (From Humason, 1972.)

For demonstrating nerve fibres as in Purkinje cells in cerebellum (*see* Fig. 16.5). Stains: neurofibrils — black; and rest of tissue — yellow/brown.

Fixation

Cut slices approximately 5 cm thick from cerebellum and place in 70% ethanol containing 0.5% glacial acetic acid for 6 h.

(1)　80% ethanol　　　　　　　　　　　　6 h
(2)　Ammoniacal alcohol (4 drops ammonia
added to 50 ml of 95% ethanol)　　　　24–36 h
(3)　Wash in distilled water, several times,
until slices sink
(4)　Pyridine (in a fume cupboard)　　　　1–2 days
(5)　Wash in running tap water overnight
(6)　Wash in distilled water, several changes

(7) Remove excess water with blotting paper

(8)* Place in large volume (80–100 ml) of 1.5% aqueous silver nitrate at 38°C in dark   5 days

(9) Rinse in distilled water

(10) Place in Cajal's reducing fluid   24 h

(11) Rinse in distilled water, several changes over at least 1 h

(12) Dehydrate and embed in wax (*see* wax infiltration and casting, section 2.1.4)

(13) Section perpendicular to organ surface— 15 μm or more thick

(14) Mount sections on slides, dry in oven, dewax in xylene and mount

Cajal's reducing fluid

Pyrogallic acid or hydroquinone	1 g
Neutral formalin	15 ml
Distilled water	100 ml

Hints

Above method gives good results with cerebellum and cerebrum of adults, but is especially good for brains of small animals. If sections not clear after (14), then treat as follows (from McClung, 1937):

(1) Bring to water

(2) Yellow chloride of gold 1 part to 500 parts water   15–30 min

(3) Rinse in water

(4) 5–10% hyposulphite of soda   30 s

(5) Water

(6) Dehydrate, clear and mount

(g) Periodic acid–Schiff technique

For visualisation of basement membranes, e.g. in kidney (*see* Fig. 12.3). Stains: basement membranes — red/purple; also stains many other substances, e.g. polysaccharides.

(1) Dewax sections, bring to water and remove mercuric chloride (*see* section 2.1.1(c)), if necessary

(2) 1% aqueous periodic acid   10 min

(3) Rinse in distilled water

(4) Stain in Schiff's reagent   10–15 min

(5) Rinse in three changes of sulphite solution   2 min each

(6) Wash in running tap water   5 min

(7) Nuclei can be counterstained in Mayer's haemalum (*see* phloxine tartrazine technique, section 2.1.7(e))   30 s

(8) Dehydrate, clear and mount

Schiff's reagent

This can be purchased already made up. An alternative is as follows:

Dissolve 1 g basic fuchsin in 200 ml boiling distilled water, stirring well. Cool to 50°C, filter and add 20 ml of 1 N HCl to filtrate. Cool, add 1 g sodium metabisulphite and stand in dark for 24 h. Then add 2 g activated charcoal and stir for 1 min. Filter and keep filtrate in dark at 0–4°C. The filtrate should now be clear and free of colour — if not, add fresh charcoal and filter. Store in glass bottle with ground stopper at 4°C. Must be colourless before use; usually stores for approximately 2 weeks.

Sulphite solution

Sodium metabisulphite (10%)	5 ml
1 N hydrochloric acid (10%)	5 ml
Distilled water	90 ml

Make up fresh each time.

(h) Modified haematoxylin and eosin method (From Elias, 1979.)

For demonstration of cartilage in, e.g., trachea (*see* Fig. 8.2) and for staining sections of whole mammalian embryos. Stains: cartilage —blue/purple; nuclei — blue/black; and cytoplasm— pink/red.

(1) Dewax sections, bring to 70% ethanol and remove mercuric chloride if necessary

(2) Stain nuclei with haematoxylin†   10–20 min

(3) Blue in tap water (weak bicarbonate solution)   5–10 min

(4) Differentiate in acid alcohol, if necessary, and repeat (3)

(5) Rinse in distilled water

(6) Counterstain either: 5 min
    (a) directly in Xylidine Ponceau (trachea)‡
       or
    place in 70% ethanol
       and then
    (b) in 0.05% alcoholic eosin†
      (whole embryo)   3–6 min

---

* Use glass bottle with ground stopper to prevent evaporation—pieces impregnated sufficiently when tobacco colour.

† *See* haematoxylin and eosin technique, section 2.1.6(a).

‡ *See* Masson's trichrome method, section 2.1.7(a).

(7)   Differentiate for (a) in 1% aqueous phosphomolybdic acid quickly and rinse in distilled water
        Differentiate for (b) in 70% ethanol
(8)   Stain in Alcian Blue (1% aqueous, filtered)   1–5 min
(9)   Rapid dehydration to absolute ethanol
(10) Clear in xylene and mount

(i)   Giemsa technique

For smears of peripheral blood and peritoneal contents. Stains: nuclei —red/purple; cytoplasm of white cells — light blue; granules of neutrophils — small and yellow/brown or red; granules of eosinophils — large and red; granules of basophils — large and purple; and erythrocytes—yellow/pink.

(1)   Thinly smear *small* drop of blood, etc., on slide, using edge of another slide for smearing
(2)   Dry *as quickly as possible* by shaking in air
(3)   Fix in absolute methanol   2 min
(4)   Stain vertically or inverted in
Giemsa stain   25–30 min
(5)   Rinse in tap water   1–2 s
(6)   Wipe off excess water
(7)   Dehydrate in tertiary butyl alcohol*   10 min
(8)   Clear in xylene and mount

Giemsa stain

    1 part of Giemsa Stock Solution (e.g. purchased from
        Gurr's, Merck, etc.)
    9 parts of buffer pH 6.8 (Gurr's buffer tablets in 100 ml
        distilled water very convenient for use)

Filter before use and make up fresh each time

2.2   HINTS FOR THE IDENTIFICATION OF HISTOLOGICAL SECTIONS

There is no magic formula which will allow the student to recognise instantly a tissue section under the microscope. There are, however, certain simple rules which will assist diagnosis.

(a)   Try to visualise three-dimensional structure

The student should always remember that histological sections examined under the microscope represent only a very small two-dimensional portion of the whole three-dimensional organ. The problem is to try to visualise the

* Usually solid at room temperature, warm slightly before use.

living three-dimensional structure from static, two-dimensional slides. Thus, for example, parallel bundles of muscle fibres will appear as long parallel rods in longitudinal section (*see* Fig. 2.1a) (so that striations can easily be seen), while in transverse section they will appear as groups of solid circles (*see* Fig. 2.1b). Since sections are rarely in perfect longitudinal or transverse planes, various intermediates between structures 2.1a and 2.1b will be seen (*see* Fig. 2.1c).

(b)   Hold it up to the light

Before placing the slide under the microscope, hold it up to the light, as this may greatly aid identification. For example, sections of kidney are (for obvious reasons!), providing the donor animal was fairly small and the section has been cut in the correct plane, kidney-shaped, which may well not be apparent under the microscope. Furthermore, gross examination will also reveal whether the tissue is solid and homogeneous, or whether it has a central cavity and is tube-like. If it is tube-like, then the section must be from the gut, reproductive, urinary, respiratory or blood vascular systems. Blood smears are also very obvious with this mode of examination.

(c)   Use the low-power objective

Next, place the section under the low-power objective (usually ×2.5, ×5 or ×10) of the microscope and note the gross morphological characteristics. For example, are there definite layers of different tissues, or cell types, arranged in regular patterns or is the tissue compact and composed mainly of one cell type (i.e. homogeneous)? If homogeneous and compact, then it is likely to be a section of a gland such as the liver, salivary gland, pancreas, etc. But *beware,* it could also be compact and through the wall, for example, of the gut or reproductive system, in which case the muscle layers present will distinguish it from most of the glands.

(d)   Use all the other objectives

Utilising all the objectives on the microscope, try to determine the main types of tissue present in the section and the relative amounts of each type. For purposes of identification of sections, the tissues in the body can be classified as follows:

Epithelial   Usually very cellular and regularly arranged in layers like bricks in a wall (Fig. 4.5d), often cover and line surfaces, may be composed of a single or many layers.

Glandular or secretory   Usually classified with epithelial but not arranged in regular layers, often forming the majority of large glands and composed of cells with large amounts of cytoplasm which are often arranged into characteristic patterns. For example, in the liver, they form the main part of the lobules and radiate out from the central vein, like the spokes in a wheel, while in the salivary glands and pancreas they are arranged into acini, like bunches of grapes around a stalk which forms the collecting duct (e.g. Figs 11.4 and 11.18).

Connective   Very variable and irregular in structure, often fibrous with few cells apparent. Forms the supporting tissue in the body and fills up the spaces between different layers or regions of an organ, e.g. submucosa of gut. Cells with very elongate nuclei (= fibroblasts) can often be seen in connective tissue (e.g. *see* submucosa in Fig. 11.8).

Muscular   Very easy to identify as they are often arranged into definite layers of pink-staining blocks of tissue. Fibrous, and in longitudinal section may show striations (under ×40 or ×100 objective) (e.g. Figs 6.1 and 6.2).

Nervous   Easily identified as they are often light staining and look very homogeneous. Contain (under high-power examination of the brain) large numbers of nerve fibres with dark-staining nuclei of the nerve cells scattered throughout the tissue (e.g. Fig. 16.4).

Lymphoid   Easily identified as they are often very darkly staining and homogeneous. Under high power they can be seen to be mainly composed of cells (= lymphocytes) with large nuclei (hence stains dark blue/black with haematoxylin) and little cytoplasm (e.g. Fig. 10.4).

Thus, if we imagine that the student has been given two specimens, A and B, to identify, by a process of elimination and utilising the above classification scheme, an intelligent answer can be arrived at:

Specimen A

(1) *By gross examination*   No definite shape, appears very uniform.

(2) *Under low power*   One cell type forms the majority of a very homogeneous tissue in which the cells are arranged in circular subunits and appear to radiate out from the centre of each subunit.

(3) *Under high power*   This confirms glandular/secretory nature of the tissue with little or no connective, muscular, nervous or lymphoid tissue present.

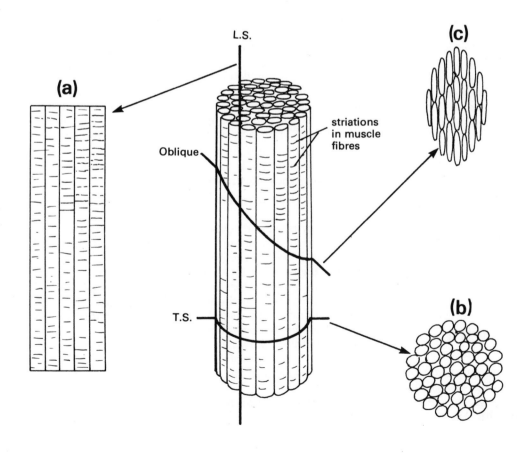

Fig. 2.1.
How a parallel bundle of muscle fibres may appear when sectioned.

(a) Longitudinal section (L.S.) — long parallel rods, striations visible.

(b) Transverse section (T.S.) — solid circles, striations not visible.

(c) Oblique section — striations not usually visible

Conclusion Liver. Cells are arranged in smaller groups in other glands such as the salivary glands or the pancreas. Lack of islets also eliminates the pancreas.

Specimen B

(1) *By gross examination* Circular outline with a hole in the centre.

(2) *Under low power* Central lumen (cavity) surrounded by 5–6 concentric layers of different types of tissue which vary from each other in thickness.

(3) *Under high power*

Layer (i)   Lines lumen, greatly infolded and formed of columnar epithelium.

Layer (ii)   Connective tissue which forms the cores of the folds and forms a thin layer below folds.

Layer (iii)   Thin muscular layer.

Layer (iv)   Amorphous connective tissue layer, containing fibres and blood vessels.

Layers (v) & (vi)   Two definite muscular layers cut in different planes.

Conclusion Composed mainly of highly infolded layers (i & ii) plus outer muscular layers (v & vi) and intervening connective tissue (iv). Probably section of gut, since, in reproductive and urinary systems, well defined layers in the muscular coat are not so obvious. The other possibility, the trachea, also has no muscular coat and many additional features. The precise region in the gut can then easily be determined by a further process of elimination, e.g. whether glands are or are not present in the connective tissue layers, the presence or absence of villi in layer (i), etc.

(e)   Examine more than one example

In most of the tissues in this book, the characteristic features are given. But the student should remember that the slides used here have been *carefully selected* to illustrate all the salient features. It is quite likely that the slide provided for study in the laboratory has only some of the characteristics listed. It is, therefore, advisable to examine more than one example of each tissue, as the preservation, staining, plane of sectioning, etc., vary greatly from one slide to another.

2.3   RECORDING OBSERVATIONS WITH DRAWINGS

Many instructors believe that there is no substitute for making accurate and clearly labelled drawings as an aid in teaching histology. By making these drawings, the student comes to appreciate the structure of the different types of tissue in the mammalian body. The drawings will also be invaluable for revision purposes.

In the example on p.35, the histological section is 60 divisions wide. The actual size of each of these divisions, and hence the width of the specimen, is then calculated by removing the histological slide from under the microscope and replacing it by a special slide (the stage micrometer) on which 0.1 mm (100 μm) and /or 0.01 mm (10 μm) subdivisions have been engraved (Fig. 2.2b). The image of the eyepiece graticule is then superimposed upon the stage micrometer (Fig. 2.2c) by focusing the objective with the coarse and fine controls. The two scales are then carefully examined until the division marks on both coincide as in Fig. 2.2c. In this drawing, each large (100 μm) division on the stage micrometer equals 20 divisions on the eyepiece graticule. Thus, in Fig. 2.2c, the distance X to Y = 100 μm on the stage micrometer and equals 20 divisions on the eyepiece graticule. Therefore each eyepiece division = 100/20 = 5 μm. Having calibrated the microscope, it is obviously very easy to calculate the size of any object placed under the same objective–eyepiece combination simply by measuring its width in units with the eyepiece graticule and multiplying this figure by 5 μm. It is, of course, necessary to calibrate the microscope only once for every objective–eyepiece combination used. Since the specimen was 60 eyepiece divisions wide, then it is 60 $\times$ 5 μm = 300 μm wide (or 0.3 mm, as we know that 1 micrometer (μm) = 0.001 mm).

Finally, if we now measure the width of our drawn specimen with a ruler, we can then calculate the actual magnification of our drawing. Thus, if in the drawing the specimen is 100 mm wide and we know from above that it is actually 0.3 mm across, then the magnification of the drawing is 100 mm/0.3 mm = $\times$ 333.

The following simple guidelines should be noted before undertaking such illustrations.

(1) It is useful to make two drawings of each tissue examined:

(i) a low-power, diagrammatic plan showing the general outline of the tissue together with the extent of the different cell layers or regions present;

(ii) a high-power ($\times$40 or $\times$100 objective) *accurate* drawing of a typical portion of the tissue. If possible, a strip 5–6 cells wide including all the different cell layers should be drawn. It is useful to indicate the location of this drawing on the low-power plan.

(2) Make these drawings on good-quality, plain, white paper with a *sharp* B or HB black lead pencil.

(3) Avoid sketching and shading. Make firm *continuous* lines.

(4) Remember, nuclei and cells are rarely empty nor are they amorphous black smudges, so indicate contents with

fine stippling.

(5) Draw large enough; tiny drawings are a waste of time. Plan your page and leave sufficient space for labelling. One drawing per page is probably adequate. Never draw on both sides of the paper.

(6) Do not waste time drawing too many cells of the same type. If a layer is 20 cells thick, draw only a few cells and indicate the remainder by a dotted line.

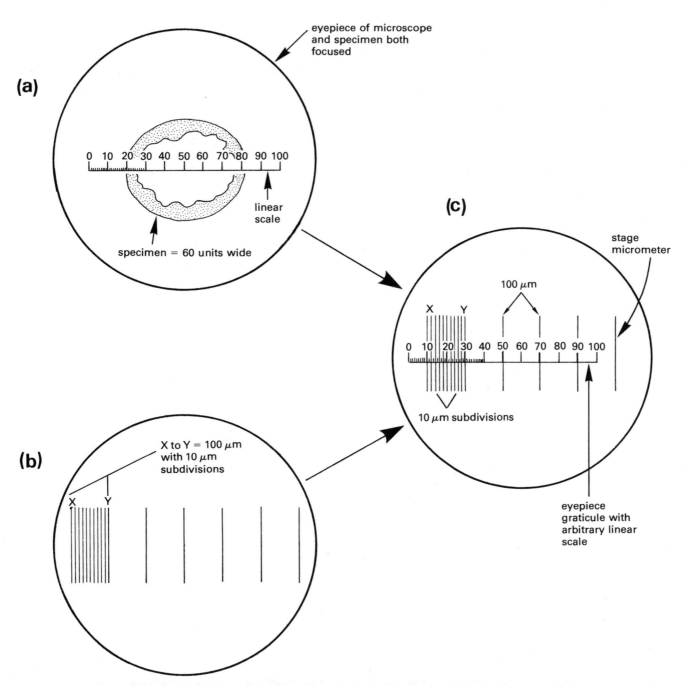

Fig. 2.2. Measurement of object size. (a) View of specimen through eyepiece graticule. (b) Stage micrometer slide (focused under normal eyepiece, i.e. one without graticule). (c) Graticule superimposed upon micrometer slide (after removal of specimen)

(7) Draw *only* what can be seen under the microscope. There is absolutely no point in copying from a textbook. If a salient feature cannot be seen, ask your instructor and/or change your slide.

(8) Remember that mitochondria, endoplasmic reticulum, Golgi, ribosomes, lysosomes, the plasma membrane, etc., are features of the cell which can only usually be seen under the electron microscope, and should *not* therefore appear in the drawings.

(9) Label the drawings clearly and accurately in black lead pencil with a ruler, using a textbook as a guide. It is also helpful to list the characteristic features of the tissue in one corner of the page.

(10) Finally, do not make the mistake of believing that the magnification of the slide under the microscope is the same as that of the drawing. Under the ×40 objective, the magnification of the drawing will certainly not be ×40 nor even ×400 (assuming a ×10 eyepiece is being used), since the final drawing will probably be at least two or three times larger than the image seen down the microscope.

The measurement of the size of the object under observation (the science of micrometry) and the magnification of the final drawing can only be made after careful calibration of the microscope. For this purpose, a small glass disc (the eyepiece graticule) engraved with an arbitrary (often linear) scale is inserted into the eyepiece* of the microscope, and the size of the object is measured in so many divisions on this scale (Fig. 2.2a).

REFERENCES

Elias, R. G. (1979) Personal communication.

Gomori, G. (1941). *Am. J. Pathol.,* **17**, 395–406.

Humason, G. L. (1972). *Animal Tissue Techniques,* 3rd edn, W. H. Freeman, San Francisco (now available as 4th edn, 1978).

McClung, C. E. (1937). *Handbook of Microscopical Technique,* 2nd edn, Oxford University Press, London.

Pantin, C. F. A. (1964). *Notes on Microscopical Technique for Zoologists,* Cambridge University Press, Cambridge.

Smith, A. and Bruton, J. (1978). *A Colour Atlas of Histological Staining Techiques,* Wolfe Medical Publications, London.

Steedman, H. F. (1960). *Section Cutting in Microscopy,* Blackwell, Oxford.

Wallington, E. A. (1972). *Histological Methods for Bone,* Butterworths, London.

* *N.B.* Special focusing eyepieces (e.g. Kellner eyepieces) for holding the graticules are available for many microscopes and should be used wherever possible in preference to the ordinary microscope eyepiece with which it may not be possible to focus the graticule sharply. The scales shown in the drawing may be very different to those on the graticule given to the student.

3 Location of Organs in Adult and Embryo

Fig. 3.1.   Adult rat showing location of main organs of the body. Note that the stomach and intestines have been displaced and are displayed to the right-hand side of the animal, and that both male and female reproductive organs are shown.

Key (with chapter numbers in parentheses):

1   eye (17)

2   tooth (11)

3   tongue (11)

4   sublingual salivary gland (11)

5   submandibular (= submaxillary) salivary gland (11)

6   parotid salivary gland (11)

7   thyroid and parathyroids covering larynx (15)

8   trachea (8)

9   thymus (10)

10   heart (muscle) (6)

11   lungs (8)

12   diaphragm

13   liver (11)

14   adrenal gland (left) (15)

15   spleen (10)

16   kidney (left) (12)

17   ureter (12)

18   posterior vena cava (= vein) (7)

19   descending aorta (= artery) (7)

20   duodenum (small intestine) (11)

21   ovary (left) (14)

22   fallopian tube (= oviduct) (14)

23   rectum (11)

24   uterus (14)

25   bladder (12)

26   tibia (long bone) (5)

27   penis (13)

28   testis (13)

29   epididymis (13)

30   vas deferens (13)

31   prostate gland (13)

32   seminal vesicle (13)

33   appendix (10) arising from caecum (11)

34   lymph nodules (10)

35   colon (large intestine) (11)

36   ileum (small intestine) (11)

37   pyloric stomach (11)

38   fundic stomach (11)

39   body wall

40   gall bladder (11)

41   pancreas (11)

42   mesentery (= connective tissue) (5)

43   hairy skin (9)

44   oesophagus (11)

45   spinal cord (16)

46   pituitary body (15)

47   cerebellum (16)

48   pineal body (15)

49   cerebrum (16)

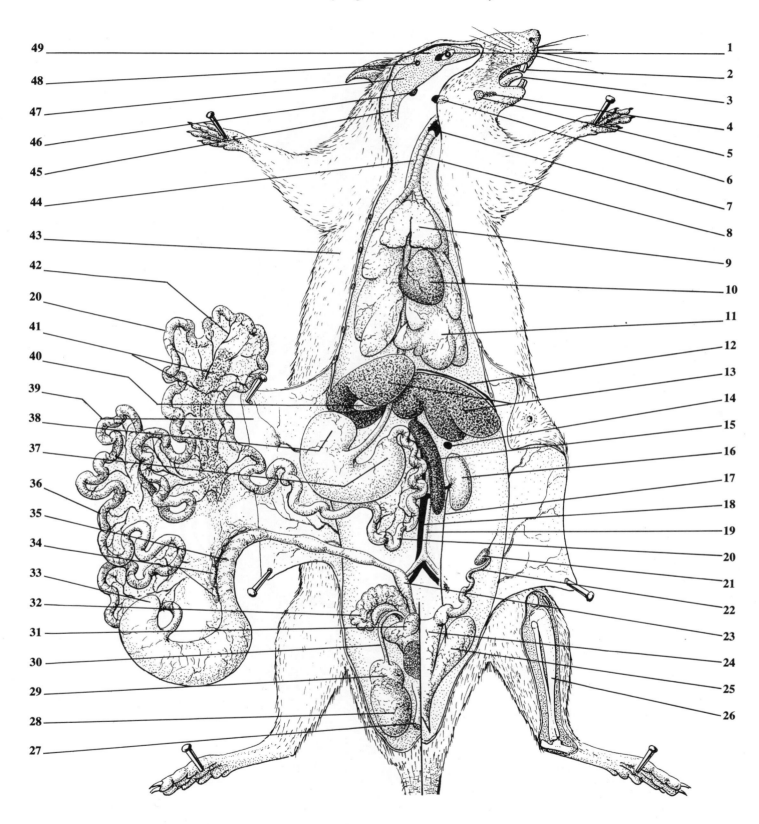

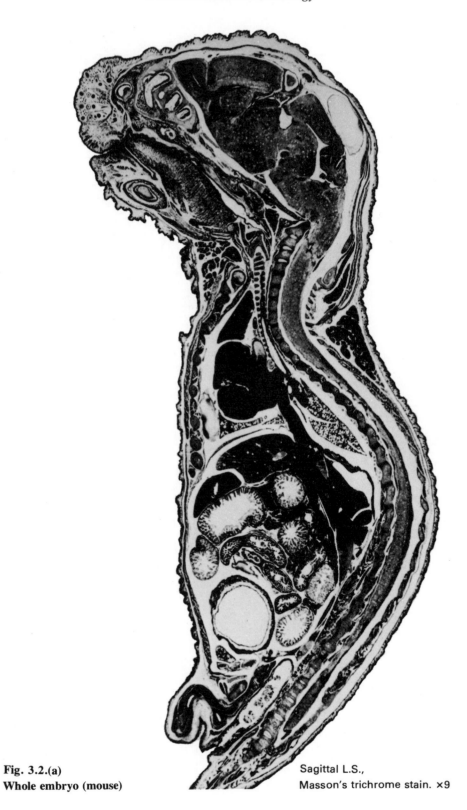

Fig. 3.2.(a)
Whole embryo (mouse)

Sagittal L.S.,
Masson's trichrome stain. ×9

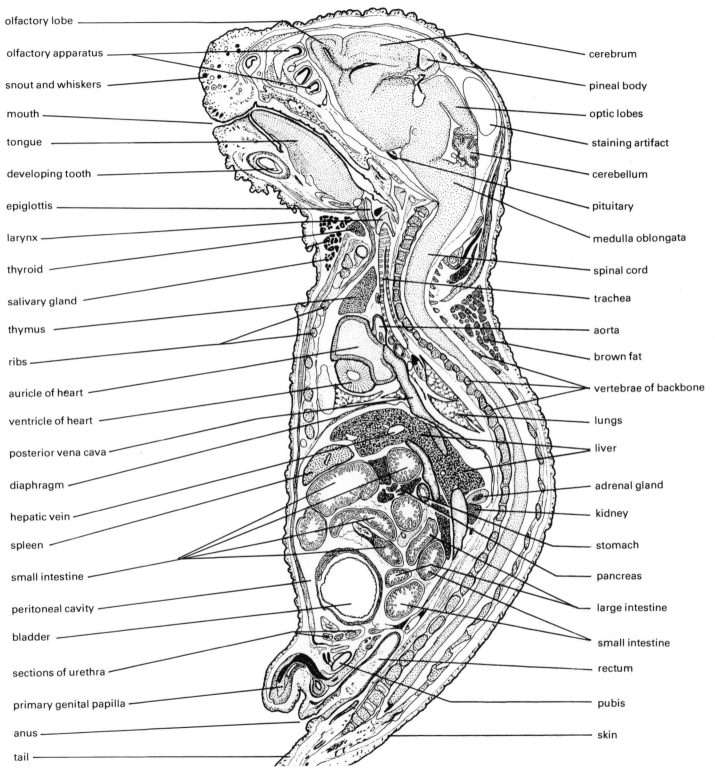

olfactory lobe

olfactory apparatus

snout and whiskers

mouth

tongue

developing tooth

epiglottis

larynx

thyroid

salivary gland

thymus

ribs

auricle of heart

ventricle of heart

posterior vena cava

diaphragm

hepatic vein

spleen

small intestine

peritoneal cavity

bladder

sections of urethra

primary genital papilla

anus

tail

cerebrum

pineal body

optic lobes

staining artifact

cerebellum

pituitary

medulla oblongata

spinal cord

trachea

aorta

brown fat

vertebrae of backbone

lungs

liver

adrenal gland

kidney

stomach

pancreas

large intestine

small intestine

rectum

pubis

skin

Fig. 3.2.(b)   Drawing of (a)

4 Epithelia

Epithelia are aggregates or sheets of closely applied cells of similar type which have very little intercellular substance, have no blood vessels and usually have high mitotic rates. Epithelia cover the outside of the body, line the body cavities, the digestive and reproductive systems and their ducts, etc., and by invagination and proliferation give rise to many different sorts of glands, e.g. salivary glands, pancreas, liver, etc. The outer surface of an epithelium is usually free (i.e. in contact with the external environment or lumen of a gland, duct, etc.), whereas the inner surface usually rests on a non-living basement membrane secreted by the epithelium and the underlying connective tissue. This arrangement is not so obvious in the case of many glands in which contact with the environment and the basement membrane may not be apparent.

4.1 CLASSIFICATION

Epithelia are usually classified according to whether they consist of one or more than one layer of cells and according to the shape of the component cells. Thus, epithelia of one cell layer are described as *simple* and those of several cell layers are *stratified* or *compound*. The shape of the cells is either *squamous* (flattened), *cuboidal* or *columnar (see* Fig. 4.1).

A single layer of flattened cells would be a *simple squamous epithelium* (as in Fig. 4.1a), while an epithelium

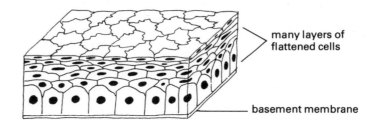

Fig. 4.2.   Stratified squamous epithelium

of several layers of flattened cells would be a *stratified squamous epithelium* (as in Fig. 4.2), and so on for the other cell shapes.

Occasionally, special names have been introduced to describe epithelia not derived from the ectoderm or endoderm, the two germ layers which give rise to most epithelia in the body. Thus the peritoneal, pleural and pericardial cavities are lined by *mesothelium,* while the blood and lymphatic vessels are lined by *endothelium.* Both of these epithelia are simple and squamous but are mesodermal in origin.

A classification scheme together with examples of the different types of epithelia is presented with the micrographs in the following pages.

4.2 FUNCTIONS

Epithelia serve many different functions and, as with all the tissues of the body, structure and function are closely

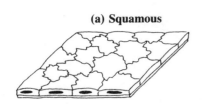

(a) Squamous

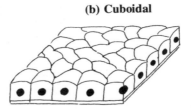

(b) Cuboidal

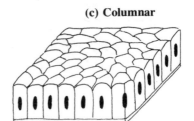

(c) Columnar

Fig. 4.1.   Cell shapes in epithelia

interrelated. Thus, on the outer surface of the body, a thick, tough, waterproof epithelium is found which is ideal for resisting mechanical stress and preventing excessive loss of vital body fluids. Histologically, this epithelium is a stratified squamous epithelium with an outer layer of dead keratinised cells. All substances entering the body and all excretory products must also pass across epithelia. The lining epithelium of the villi of the small intestine is simple and columnar in form, and the free surface of each columnar cell has a so-called *striated border* that consists of numerous small projections or microvilli (not usually visible in light microscopy) which increase the surface area for absorption of nutrients. Epithelia are specialised for numerous other functions such as: sensory reception, e.g. taste buds in the tongue; synthesis of proteins, hormones, mucus, etc., in various glands; movement of substances by

means of cilia on their free surfaces, e.g. nasal mucosa, trachea, etc.; storage of large volumes of waste products, as with the transitional epithelium lining the bladder, etc.

4.3   EXOCRINE AND ENDOCRINE GLANDS

As mentioned above, many glands are formed by invagination from epithelia and subsequent proliferation and differentiation (but not all, e.g. corpus luteum, which is formed in the ovary from connective tissue). If the gland retains its connection to the outside surface, this subsequently forms the main duct of the gland and serves to discharge the products of secretion. Such glands are called *exocrine glands* and include the salivary gland, pancreas, liver, etc. (Fig. 4.3a) If the epithelial ducts are lost (so that

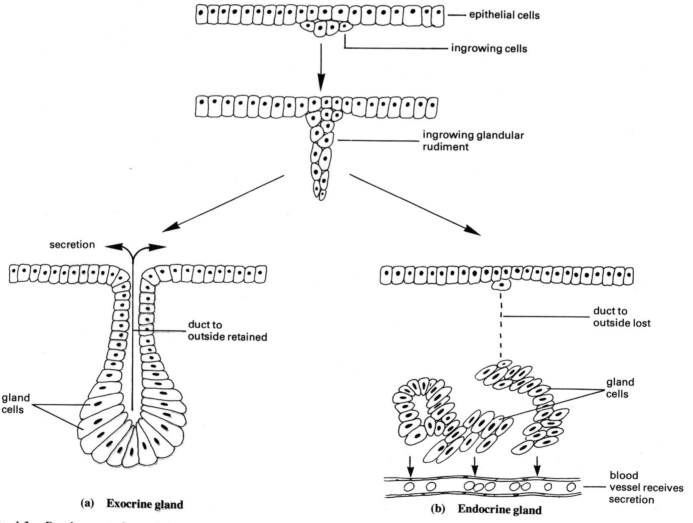

(a)   Exocrine gland

(b)   Endocrine gland

Fig. 4.3.   Development of exocrine and endocrine glands

the gland no longer discharges its products to the outer surface with which it now has no connection), then the gland is termed an *endocrine gland* or *ductless gland* (Fig. 4.3b). Endocrine glands include all the hormone-producing glands, e.g. pituitary, etc., and they discharge their products *directly* into the bloodstream.

Exocrine glands themselves are also classified depending upon the amount of branching that the ducts undergo and according to the shape of the secretory portion of the gland itself. Thus, if the duct remains unbranched and the cells form a simple invaginated tube, e.g. crypts of Lieberkühn, then this is a *simple tubular gland* (Fig. 4.4a). If, on the other hand, the duct branches but the secretory part remains tubular, this is a *compound tubular gland* (Fig. 4.4b), e.g. some of the Brunner's glands of the duodenum.

Other categories include simple and compound alveolar (= acinar) glands, in which the secretory portion is expanded and sac-like; coiled and branched tubular glands; and mixed glands containing both tubular and alveolar components.

Figure 4.5 shows micrographs of different types of epithelia.

(a) Simple tubular gland

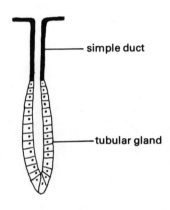

simple duct

tubular gland

(b) Compound tubular gland

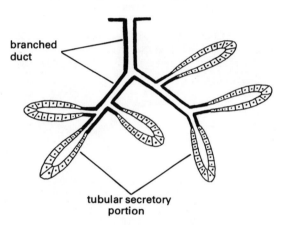

branched duct

tubular secretory portion

Fig. 4.4. Two types of exocrine glands

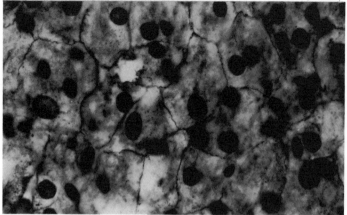

Fig. 4.5.(a)   Simple squamous epithelium (mesentery, mammal), whole mount, silver stain. ×450

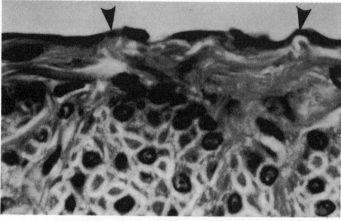

Fig. 4.5.(b)   Simple squamous epithelium (arrowheads) (fallopian tube, rabbit), T.S. ×1100

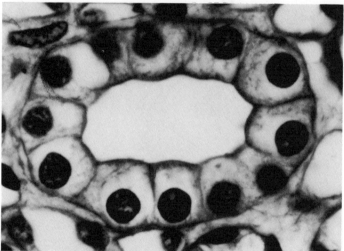

Fig. 4.5.(c)   Simple cuboidal epithelium (collecting tubule in medulla of kidney, rabbit), T.S. ×1400

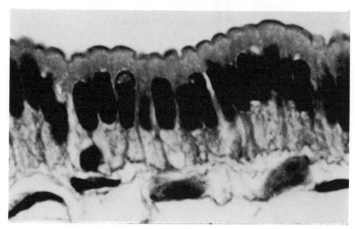

Fig. 4.5.(d)   Simple columnar epithelium (gall bladder, rabbit), section. ×1100

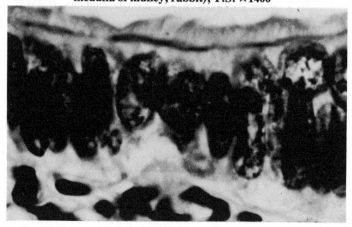

Fig. 4.5.(e)   Simple ciliated columnar epithelium (fallopian tube, rabbit), T.S. ×1500

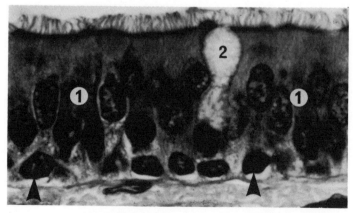

Fig. 4.5.(f)   Pseudostratified ciliated columnar epithelium (trachea, sheep). Note columnar cells (1), goblet cells (2) and basal cells (arrowheads). T.S. ×1200

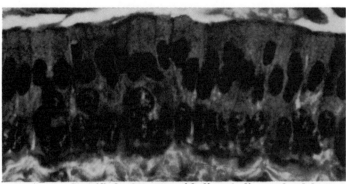

Fig. 4.5.(g) Stratified columnar epithelium (salivary gland duct, mammal), T.S. ×1100

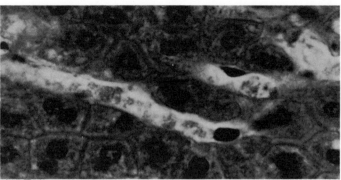

Fig. 4.5.(h) Glandular epithelium (cuboidal cells of liver, rat), section. ×800

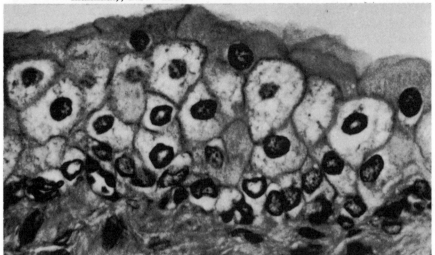

Fig. 4.5.(i) Stratified transitional epithelium (bladder, rabbit), section. ×650

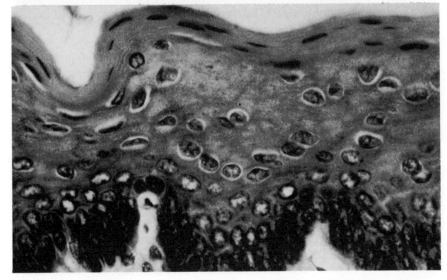

Fig. 4.5.(j) Stratified squamous epithelium (oesophagus, rabbit), T.S. ×700

Classification

1. *Simple* (single layer of cells)
(i) Squamous, e.g. mesenteries, lining of blood vessels, serosa of gut and fallopian tube, wall of Bowman's capsule, etc. (*see* Figs 4.5(a) and (b))
(ii) Cuboidal, e.g. wall of ovary, kidney tubules, etc. (*see* Fig. 4.5(c))
(iii) Columnar, e.g. villi of gut, gall bladder; often ciliated as in fallopian tube (*see* Figs 4.5(d) and (e))

2. *Pseudostratified* (also single layer of cells but appears multilayered)
(i) Columnar, e.g. epididymis, prostate; often ciliated as in trachea (*see* Fig. 4.5(f))

3. *Stratified* (many layers of cells)
(i) Squamous, e.g. oesophagus, vagina (*see* Fig. 4.5(j))
(ii) Transitional, e.g. bladder, ureters; found where urine stored and discharged and varies in structure according to whether or not stretched by urine present; many cell layers thick in collapsed or contracted state and only 2–3 layers in distended state (*see* Fig. 4.5(i) = collapsed state)
(iii) Columnar, e.g. large ducts of salivary glands, soft palate, etc. (*see* Fig.4.5(g))

N.B. Glands are composed of large numbers of cells of simple columnar or cuboidal epithelia or even those of other epithelial type (*see* Fig.4.5(h))

5 Connective and Supporting Tissues

As the name suggests, connective tissue interconnects the various parts of the body, and at the same time it also has a vital supportive role. Connective tissues are found throughout the animal and differ greatly in structure from one region to another. All connective tissues, however, consist basically of cells scattered in a large amount of extracellular material (= matrix) secreted by them which may be fluid, semi-solid or solid, and usually contains fibrous material of different kinds. The nature and distribution of the component cells and matrix are used as a basis for classifying connective tissues.

5.1 CLASSIFICATION

Fluid matrix

Blood and haemopoietic tissue — *see* Chapter 7.

Semi-solid matrix with fibres

Areolar or loose connective tissue
Dense connective tissue
Regular connective tissue (tendon)
Elastic tissue
Reticular tissue
Adipose tissue

Solid matrix

Cartilage
Bone

All these types of connective tissue arise from mesenchyme cells which are derivatives of embryonic mesoderm.

5.2 DESCRIPTION

5.2.1 Areolar or loose connective tissue

Such tissue (Fig. 5.1) consists of an amorphous, semi-solid matrix containing proteinaceous fibrous material and various types of cells scattered at random. The amorphous matrix is composed of *mucopolysaccharides* (= glycosaminoglycans), such as hyaluronic acid. The fibres include a few *elastic fibres* and bundles of *collagen* and these greatly strengthen the tissue. The cells include fibroblasts, fixed macrophages (= histiocytes) and mast cells.

Fibroblasts are responsible for synthesis and secretion of the amorphous matrix and the proteinaceous fibres. They are often spindle-shaped or stellate (star-shaped) with an elongate nucleus, and collagen precursors (= tropocollagen) are synthesised within the cell and passed to the outside where they polymerise to form collagen.

Fixed macrophages often appear similar in structure to fibroblasts and may be as common. They also tend to spread out and put out cytoplasmic extensions with which they are capable of ingesting *(phagocytosing)* large numbers of foreign microbes. Fixed macrophages are thus important in the cellular defence against invading bacteria, etc.

Mast cells are the third cell type found in areolar tissue *(see* Fig. 7.1) and they are large in rats but small in man. The nucleus is often masked by the large numbers of cytoplasmic granules present. These granules contain pharmacologically active substances such as heparin and histamine which function during inflammatory or allergic reactions.

Areolar or loose connective tissue is present throughout the body and forms the packing between organs and tissues, and it is usually deposited in thin sheets around glands, nerves, blood vessels and underneath epithelia, etc.

5.2.2 Dense connective tissue

This consists of large numbers of *randomly* arranged *bundles of collagen* fibres which fill the ground substance and form a dense tissue. Elastic fibres may also be quite common. The cells present are mainly fibroblasts, although macrophages are found. This tissue forms the majority of the dermis *(see* Figs 9.1 and 9.2), and the capsules and sheaths around glands (e.g. Fig. 15.4), nerves, etc. Intermediates between areolar tissue and dense connective tissue are found and vary in the amount of collagen deposited.

5.2.3 Regular connective tissue

Regular connective tissue (Fig. 5.2) is similar to dense connective tissue except that the *collagen bundles* are very *closely packed* and are parallel to each other. The only cells present are extremely *elongate fibroblasts* which form in rows between the bundles of collagen. Elastic fibres may also be present. Regular connective tissue has great strength, is usually ensheathed by dense connective tissue and is found in the tendons, ligaments, cornea, etc.

5.2.4 Elastic tissue

This is also a form of dense connective tissue in which there is a preponderance of elastic fibres, so that the tissue is strong but flexible. Elastic tissue is found in the walls of large arteries (Fig. 7.3), the trachea, bronchi, etc.

5.2.5 Reticular tissue

This is composed of reticular fibres which do not stain in haematoxylin and eosin preparations. Reticular fibres are also proteinaceous and are closely related to collagen, except that they are very fine and form delicate supportive networks in lymphoid tissue, e.g. spleen and haemopoietic tissue (particularly the bone marrow). There are usually fibroblasts and phagocytic macrophages present.

5.2.6 Adipose tissue

Adipose tissue (Fig. 5.3) consists of cells filled with *stores of fat* supported by fine fibres of collagen. There is usually a rich blood supply. The fat droplets usually fill the cells and displace the nucleus and cytoplasm to the edge of the cell, so that they may be difficult to see. There are two types of adipose tissue, designated *white* and *brown,* which differ in their appearance, distribution and utilisation by the body. White adipose tissue is widely distributed and is common in the subcutaneous tissues, while brown fat is concentrated in definite regions in the body such as between the shoulder blades. Both types of fat act as energy stores which can be utilised or built up under the direction of certain hormones.

5.2.7 Cartilage

Cartilage (Fig. 5.4) is a special type of connective tissue which has a supportive role in the body. It contains cells of only one type, the *chondrocytes,* which are scattered throughout a solid matrix composed mainly of a sulphated mucopolysaccharide, *chondroitin sulphate*. The matrix is also strengthened by *collagen fibres* which are difficult to discern in ordinary histological preparations under the light microscope. The chondrocytes lie in small spaces called *lacunae* and secrete the intercellular substances of the matrix. The whole of the cartilage is enclosed in a sheath, the *perichondrium,* except at points of articulation, such as in the joints, where cartilage covers and protects the apposed bones. The perichondrium usually consists of an outer fibroblast layer and an inner layer of transitional cells which are transforming into chondrocytes.

Three types of cartilage are generally recognised, namely hyaline cartilage, elastic cartilage and fibrocartilage, and they differ in the nature of their matrices.

Hyaline cartilage is the most common and is found widely distributed in the foetal skeleton, and also occurs in the adult on the surfaces of the joints and in the nose, and forms the cartilaginous rings in the trachea, larynx and bronchi. It is clear and often has a bluish/white appearance. Hyaline cartilage forms the template for a common type of bone formation called *endochondral ossification* (*see* Figs 5.5 and 5.6), during which the chondrocytes enlarge, and the cartilage becomes calcified and broken down and is replaced by bone laid down by *osteoblasts*.

Elastic cartilage is similar to hyaline cartilage except that the matrix contains large numbers of elastic fibres which, of course, increase the elasticity of this tissue. It is the least common type of cartilage and is found in the external ear, the auditory and eustachian tubes, the epiglottis and parts of the larynx.

Fibrocartilage is also like hyaline cartilage except for the presence of additional collagen fibres in its matrix. It thus has great strength and is found in the intervertebral discs, in the symphysis pubis, and in the attachments of tendons to bones.

5.2.8 Bone

Like cartilage, bone (Figs 5.5–5.7) is a special type of connective tissue with a supportive function. It also consists of cells enclosed in lacunae and scattered in a matrix containing collagen fibres. However, bone differs from cartilage in that the matrix becomes *calcified* and yet the tissue *remains viable*. This is because the cells (= *osteocytes*) in bone tissue are interconnected by tiny tubules, called *canaliculi,* which allow the vital nutrients to diffuse from the numerous blood vessels and so reach the cells. The actual matrix of bone is laid down by *osteoblasts* that originate from the *periosteum* which surrounds the bony tissue. Like the perichondrium of cartilage, the periosteum consists of an outer fibrous layer and an inner layer of cells which generate the osteoblasts.

Two types of bone, namely *spongy bone* (= *membrane or cancellous bone*) and *compact bone,* are recognised, and both types can be observed in a long bone such as the femur. The *epiphyses* (= swollen ends of a long bone) at each end of the *diaphysis* (= shaft) are composed mainly of spongy bone, while the diaphysis consists of a hollow tube of compact bone enclosing the *bone marrow.* Spongy bone consists of numerous rods or plates of bone, called *trabeculae,* separated by a system of wide interconnecting spaces often containing bone marrow. In contrast, compact bone, as the name suggests, is solid and without any interconnecting spaces. Both of these types of bone, however, have a similar microscopic structure, and are composed of cylindrical subunits termed *osteons* or *Haversian systems.* Each osteon is composed of concentric layers or *lamellae* of bone, very much like the growth rings in the trunk of a tree. The whole structure is perforated by numerous lacunae containing the osteocytes which communicate by means of the canaliculi, through which nutrient passes to the cells via a central blood vessel in the 'hub' or *Haversian canal* of each osteon (*see* Fig. 5.7).

Ossification (or bone formation) takes place by one of two ways:
(1) by utilising a *hyaline cartilage template* on which to lay down the bony material = *endochondral ossification* (*see* Figs 5.5 and 5.6), e.g. long bones, vertebrae, etc.;
(2) by utilising *mesenchyme cells* which come together and form a *membranous structure* containing osteoblasts which lay down bone and form centres for ossification = *intramembranous ossification,* e.g. many of the flat bones in the skull.

Finally, bone is not a static tissue but is consistently being remodelled during growth. This reshaping of bone is achieved by an interplay of *bone resorption* by large multinucleate *osteoclasts* and new bone formation by the osteoblasts.

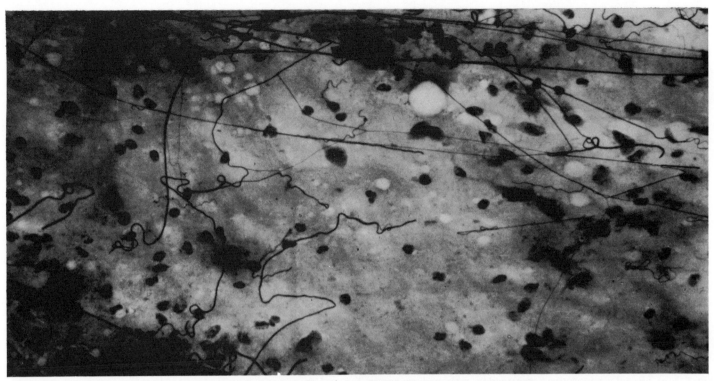

Fig. 5.1.(a) **Areolar or loose connective tissue (subcutaneous, rat), medium power, whole mount. ×350**

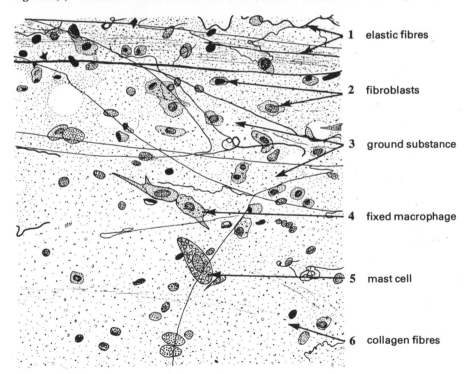

1 elastic fibres

2 fibroblasts

3 ground substance

4 fixed macrophage

5 mast cell

6 collagen fibres

Fig. 5.1.(b) **Drawing of right-hand side of (a)**

Characteristic features of areolar connective tissue

(A)   Many fibres of different sorts interwoven within tissue

(B)   No regular arrangement of components and largely amorphous

(C)   Contains numerous white blood cells and fibroblasts scattered singly throughout

Functions

(A)   Binds tissues together and protects them

(B)   The white cells (macrophages and mast cells) defend the body against invading microbes by phagocytosis and by the release of pharmacologically active substances (from mast cells)

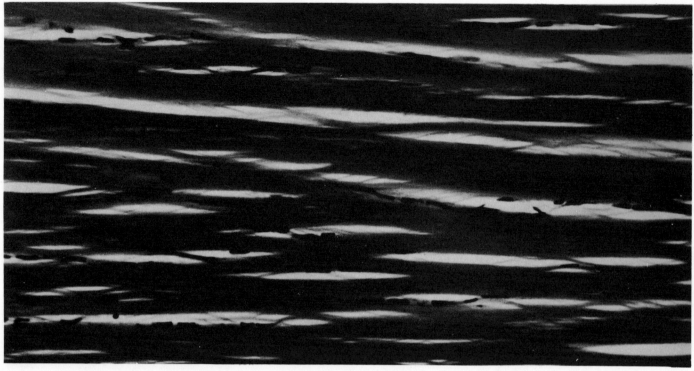

Fig. 5.2.(a)   Regular connective tissue (tendon, rat), medium power. L.S. ×450

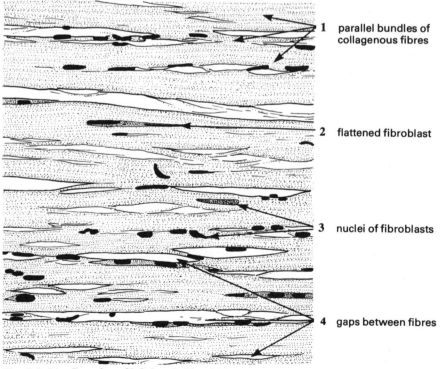

1 parallel bundles of
      collagenous fibres

2 flattened fibroblast

3 nuclei of fibroblasts

4 gaps between fibres

Fig. 5.2.(b)   Drawing of left-hand side of (a)

*Characteristic features of regular
connective tissue*

(A)   Composed of parallel, amorphous
fibres separated by rows of flattened
cells

(B)   In contrast to striped and cardiac
muscle, no striations present, and unlike
cardiac muscle, individual fibres are
unbranched

(C)   Rows of fibroblasts between
fibres distinguish tendon from smooth
muscle which it superficially resembles

(D)   Structure similar to ligament

Functions

(A)   Attaches muscles to bones

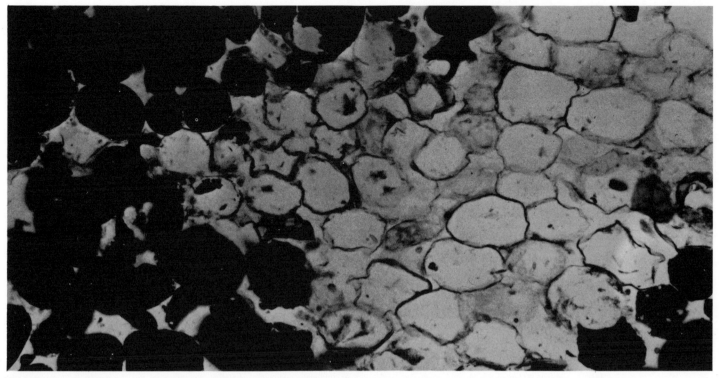

Fig. 5.3.(a)   Adipose tissue (mammal), medium-power section, treated with osmium tetroxide to stain fat black. ×350

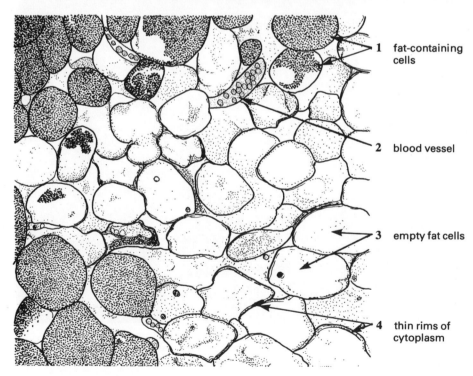

1 fat-containing cells

2 blood vessel

3 empty fat cells

4 thin rims of cytoplasm

Fig. 5.3.(b)   Drawing of central portion of (a)

Characteristic features of adipose tissue

(A)   Composed of numerous, round, often empty, cells in which the cytoplasm and nucleus are confined to a thin peripheral rim

(B)   Fat is usually extracted by the solvents used during tissue preparation but can be preserved in some of the fat cells by prior fixation in osmium tetroxide (see micrograph (a)), after which it appears uniformly black

(C)   Fat cells often arranged into groups by connective tissue strands (not shown in (a))

(D)   Do not confuse with lung, which is ramified by numerous ducts, tubes and blood vessels

Functions

(A)   Stores fat, which is broken down and used for energy production

(B)   Insulates body against cold

(C)   Protects vital organs

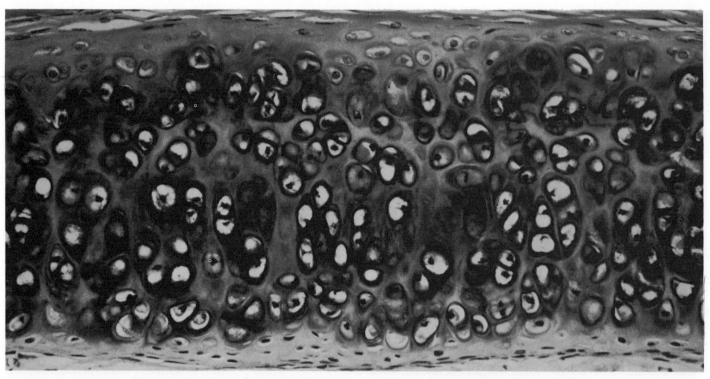

Fig. 5.4.(a)   Hyaline cartilage (trachea, rat), medium-power section, Alcian Blue and haematoxylin stain. ×360

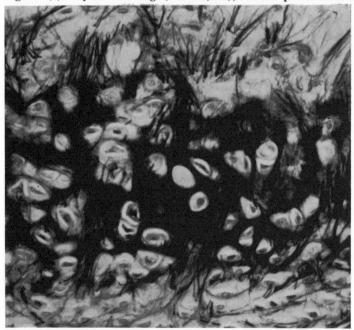

Fig. 5.4.(b)   Elastic cartilage (epiglottis, mammal), medium-power section showing bundles of elastic fibres in the matrix between cells. Special stain (e.g. Verhoeff's elastin stain) to show up elastic fibres. ×330

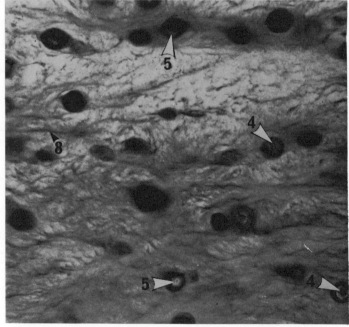

Fig. 5.4.(c)   Fibrocartilage (pubic symphysis, mammal), medium-power section showing bundles of collagen fibres (8) between chondrocytes (4). Lacunae (5). ×300

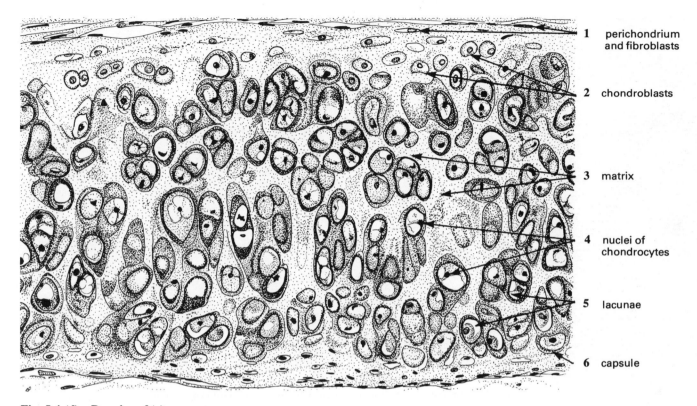

1 perichondrium and fibroblasts

2 chondroblasts

3 matrix

4 nuclei of chondrocytes

5 lacunae

6 capsule

Fig. 5.4.(d)   Drawing of (a)

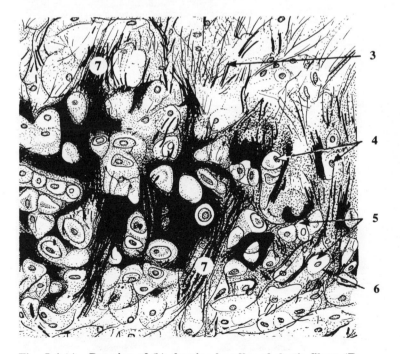

3

4

5

6

Fig. 5.4.(e)   Drawing of (b) showing bundles of elastic fibres (7)

Characteristic features of cartilage

(A)   Composed of small groups of cells embedded in a fibrous matrix

(B)   Cells rest in small spaces called lacunae

(C)   No muscles or nerves present

Functions

(A)   Supports tissues, e.g. trachea, nose, etc.

(B)   Covers and protects ends of joints, between vertebrae, etc.

(C)   Forms much of embryonic skeleton and allows growth in length of bones

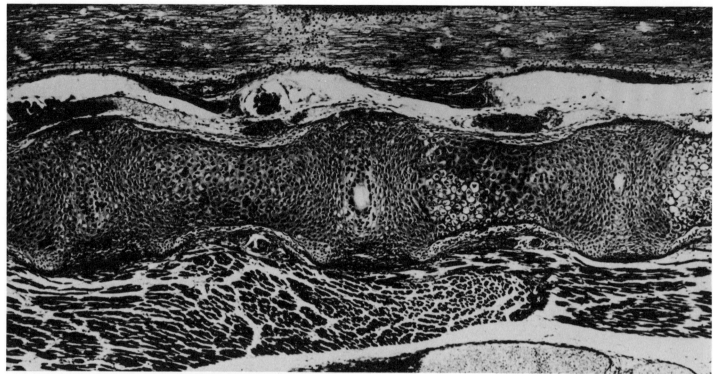

Fig. 5.5.(a)   Early stage in ossification (endochondral bone formation) in vertebral column (rat, embryo) showing undifferentiated hyaline cartilage model. Section. ×90

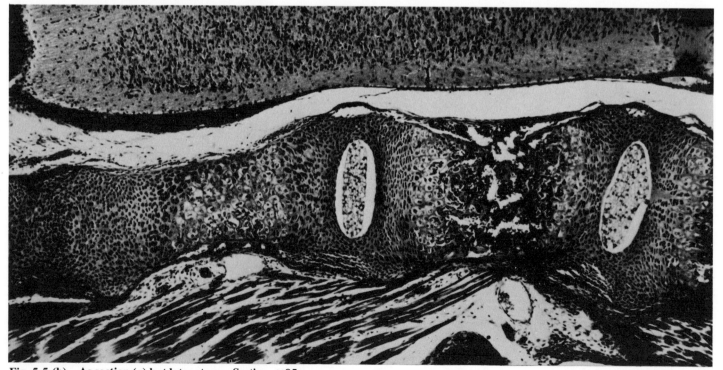

Fig. 5.5.(b)   As section (a) but later stages. Section. ×95

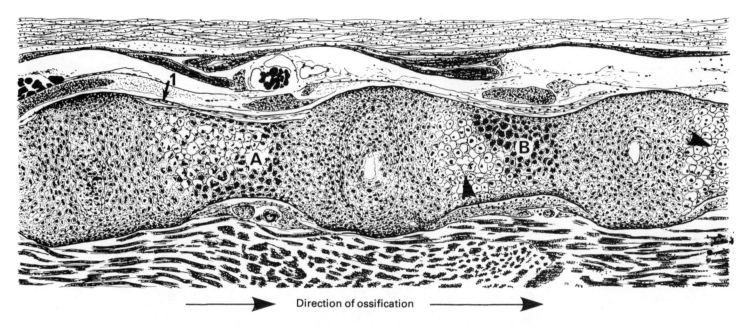

Direction of ossification

Fig. 5.5.(c)　Drawing of (a) showing undifferentiated hyaline cartilage model (A). Note perichondrium (1) and regions of hypertrophy (enlargement) of chondrocytes (arrowheads) and their calcification to stain deeply (B) which represent first stages in development of centres of endochondral ossification

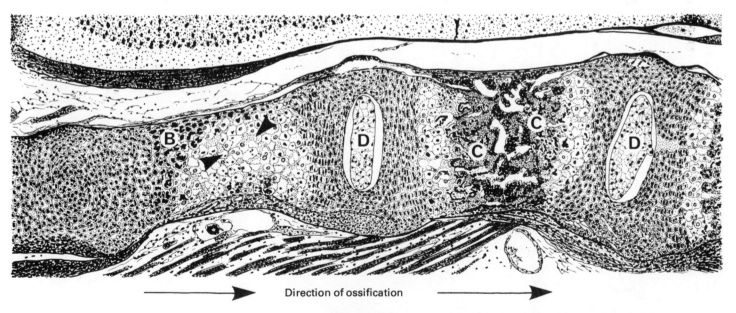

Direction of ossification

Fig. 5.5.(d)　Drawing of (b). Hypertrophy of chondrocytes (arrowheads) and calcification of matrix (B) continue and the calcified cartilage breaks down to become invaded by osteoblasts which lay down trabeculae of bone (C). Note intervertebral discs (D)

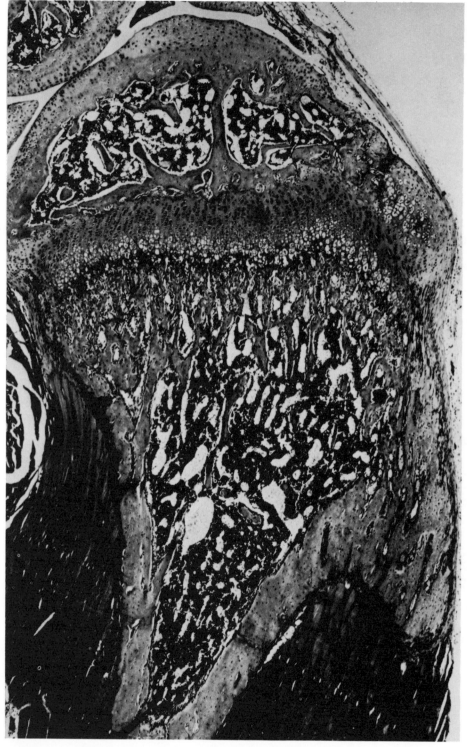

Fig. 5.6.(a)   Tibia (mouse), upper end showing ossification of the diaphysis and upper epiphysis. Low-power section. ×60

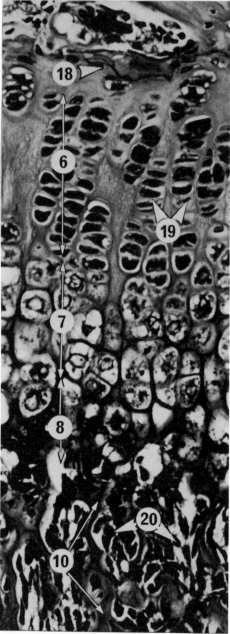

Fig. 5.6.(b)   Tibia (mouse), medium power of epiphyseal plate (boxed area in (c)). Note zones of resting cartilage (18), proliferating cartilage (6), hypertrophying cartilage (7) and calcifying cartilage (8), and columns of chondrocytes (19), osteoblasts (20) and bony trabeculae in metaphysis (10). ×400

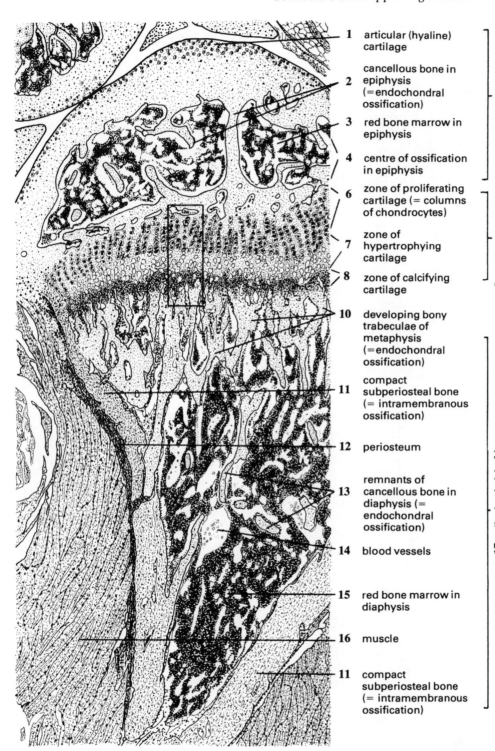

1   articular (hyaline) cartilage

2   cancellous bone in epiphysis (=endochondral ossification)

3   red bone marrow in epiphysis

4   centre of ossification in epiphysis

5   epiphysis

6   zone of proliferating cartilage (= columns of chondrocytes)

7   zone of hypertrophying cartilage

8   zone of calcifying cartilage

9   epiphyseal plate

10   developing bony trabeculae of metaphysis (=endochondral ossification)

11   compact subperiosteal bone (= intramembranous ossification)

12   periosteum

13   remnants of cancellous bone in diaphysis (= endochondral ossification)

14   blood vessels

15   red bone marrow in diaphysis

16   muscle

17   diaphysis (shaft)

11   compact subperiosteal bone (= intramembranous ossification)

Fig. 5.6.(c)   Drawing of left-hand side of (a)

Outline of ossification of a long bone

First, a cartilage template or model develops and becomes surrounded by a membrane (= perichondrium) from which further chondrocytes develop. The chondrocytes in the midpart of the model hypertrophy (enlarge) and synthesise phosphatase which calcifies the matrix. Calcification kills the chondrocytes and the cartilage breaks down to leave gaps. Meanwhile, the perichondrium becomes vascularised and develops into the periosteum which contains osteoblasts and osteocytes which form a thin shell of subperiosteal bone around the template (= intramembranous ossification). Osteoblasts from this shell move into the central degenerating cartilage and lay down bony trabeculae (= cancellous bone) on the cartilaginous remnants (= endochondral ossification). Bone formation then proceeds from this diaphyseal centre of ossification towards each end and a marrow cavity develops. The epiphyseal centres of ossification develop (also = endochondral ossification) only after ossification of the diaphysis (= shaft) is well advanced. Eventually the bone of the epiphyses and diaphysis are only separated by a plate of cartilage (= epiphyseal plate) which allows for increase in length of the bone. This plate then disappears and bone growth ceases although mature bones are consistently remodelled by resorption (by osteoclasts) and deposition of bone (by osteoblasts). In long bones, some of the cancellous bone is converted to compact bone by deposition of layers of bone on the surfaces of the trabeculae so that spaces between these are reduced. Compact bone usually forms a hollow cylinder in the subperiosteal region of the diaphysis and encloses cancellous bone and marrow. The epiphyses are mainly composed of cancellous bone

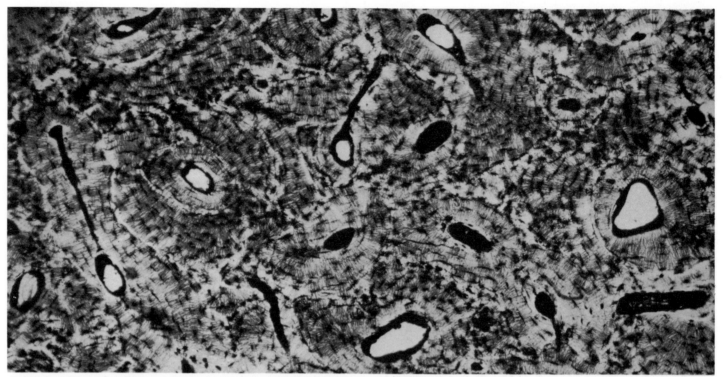

Fig. 5.7.(a)   Compact bone (human), low power, ground T.S., stained with Indian Ink. ×110

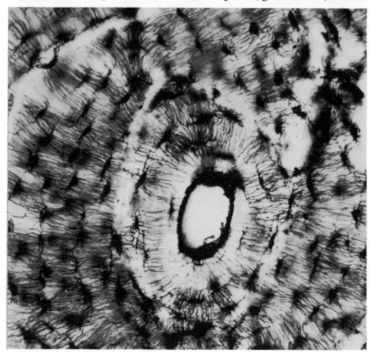

Fig. 5.7.(b)   Compact bone (human), medium power of a
               Haversian system, ground T.S., stained with Indian
               Ink. ×280

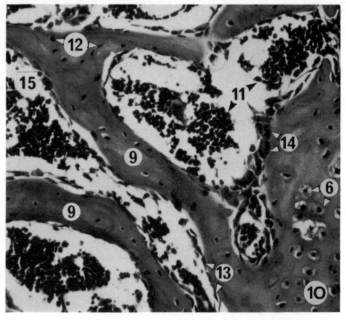

Fig. 5.7.(c)   Spongy bone (= cancellous bone) (greyhound,
               knee), medium-power section. Note trabeculae
               (9), hyaline cartilage (10) for articulation, red
               bone marrow (11), osteocytes (12), osteoblasts
               (13), osteoclasts (14) and lacunae (6). × 250

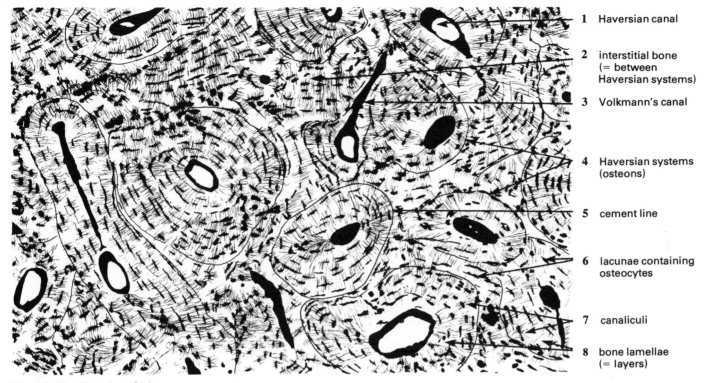

1 Haversian canal

2 interstitial bone (= between Haversian systems)

3 Volkmann's canal

4 Haversian systems (osteons)

5 cement line

6 lacunae containing osteocytes

7 canaliculi

8 bone lamellae (= layers)

Fig. 5.7.(d)   Drawing of (a)

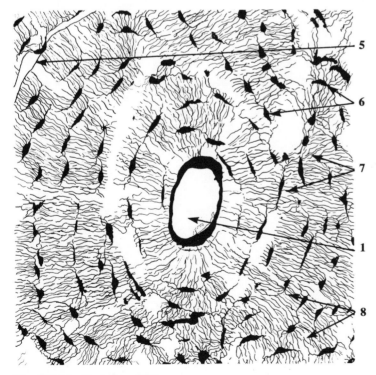

Fig. 5.7.(e)   Drawing of (b)

Characteristic features of bone

(A)   Compact bone is solid and consists of numerous cylindrical structures (= Haversian systems) which in cross section appear like tree trunks with concentric growth rings (= lamellae). Each Haversian system is ramified by a complex system of fine canals and lacunae

(B)   Spongy bone consists of many small interconnecting bars of tissue (= trabeculae) enclosing spaces containing darkly staining cell masses (= bone marrow)

Functions

(A)   Supports body and forms skeleton for movement, protection, etc.

(B)   Spongy bone forms a template in skull, etc., for laying down of compact bone

(C)   Stores calcium and phosphorus

(D)   Encloses haemopoietic (= blood-forming) tissue = bone marrow

6 Muscular Tissues

Muscles are responsible for movements of the body and organs, and are composed of elongated cells called fibres. Movements result from contraction of these fibres, between which are found connective tissue, blood vessels and nerves. Three types of muscle are recognised:

Striped muscle (= striated, skeletal or voluntary muscle)
Cardiac muscle
Smooth muscle (= involuntary muscle)

6.1 STRIPED MUSCLE

Striped muscle (Fig. 6.1) consists of very long fibres (= cells) each containing many nuclei which are located at the periphery of the fibres. The cytoplasm of each fibre contains many longitudinally orientated *myofibrils* each consisting of alternating light and dark regions which are in line with those of adjacent myofibrils, thus imparting the striped appearance to the fibres. Striped muscle is also called *voluntary muscle,* as it is under control of the conscious mind and contracts in response to motor impulses from the brain or spinal cord.

Striped muscle is responsible for *rapid contractions* over relatively short periods and forms the majority of the 'red meat' of the body. It is found attached by tendons to the skeleton (hence the term *skeletal muscle*) and produces all the movements of the body. It is also found in the diaphragm, face, eyes, ears, etc.

6.2 CARDIAC MUSCLE

As the name implies, cardiac muscle (Fig. 6.2) is confined to the heart, and like striped muscle consists of fibres or cells with cross-striations. In contrast to striped muscle, however, there is usually a single centrally located nucleus per fibre, and the fibres *branch* and interconnect with each other. Furthermore, the fibres are joined end to end by transverse, darkly staining bands called *intercalated discs.* Cardiac muscle, like smooth muscle, is not under direct conscious control and is innervated by the autonomic nervous system. Contractions are, however, *rapid* and *rhythmic.*

6.3 SMOOTH MUSCLE

Smooth muscle (Fig. 6.3) is composed of bundles of spindle-shaped cells or fibres which show no cross-striations or branches and have a central nucleus. Special staining techniques may reveal the presence of longitudinal fibrils called myofibrils, which are present in each cell and are responsible for contraction. Smooth muscle is also called *involuntary muscle* as it is not under the control of the conscious mind and is innervated by the autonomic nervous system.

Smooth muscle is responsible for relatively *slow contractions* over long periods and is found in the walls of many tubular organs. The wall of the digestive tube has two layers of smooth muscle which produce waves of contraction (= *peristalsis*) which move the food along the gut. The contractions of the uterus during labour are induced by layers of smooth muscle in the uterine wall. Smooth muscle is also located in the walls of the blood vessels (alters blood pressure), the respiratory bronchi and bronchioles (can induce asthma), the genital and urinary tracts, the skin (elevates the hair), the mammary gland, the eye, etc.

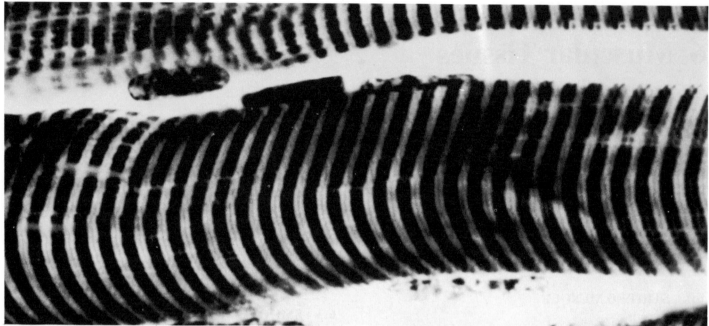

Fig. 6.1.(a)   Striped muscle (human, tongue), L.S., high power showing characteristic banding (= striations). Iron haematoxylin stain. ×2500

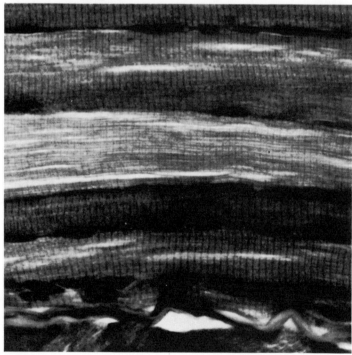

Fig. 6.1.(b)   Striped muscle fibres (rabbit, tongue), L.S., high power showing less intense appearance of banding after haematoxylin and eosin staining. ×930

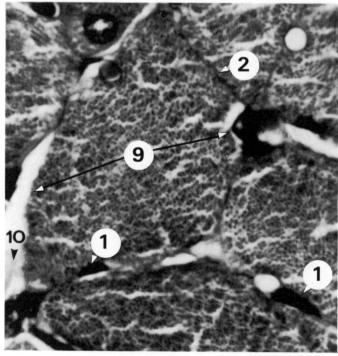

Fig. 6.1.(c)   Striped muscle (rabbit, tongue) T.S., high power. Note polygonal groups (Cohnheim fields) (9) of myofibrils, peripheral nuclei (1), position of sarcolemma (2) and connective tissue (10) in gaps produced during processing. ×2000

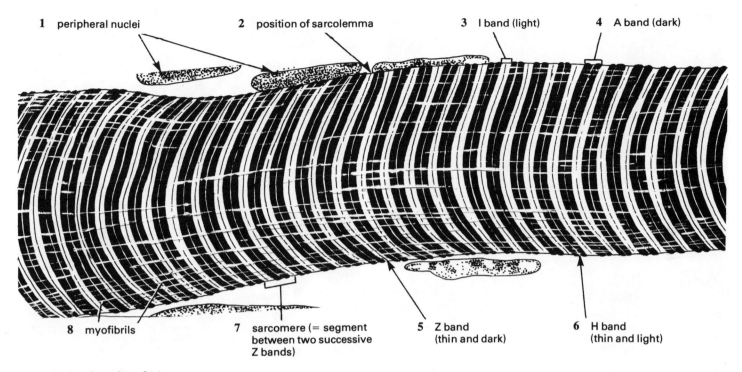

1 peripheral nuclei   2 position of sarcolemma   3 I band (light)   4 A band (dark)

8 myofibrils

7 sarcomere (= segment between two successive Z bands)

5 Z band (thin and dark)

6 H band (thin and light)

Fig. 6.1.(d) Drawing of (a)

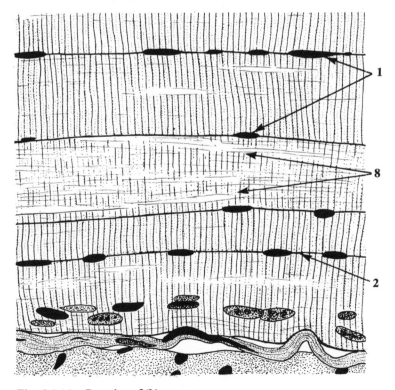

Fig. 6.1.(e) Drawing of (b)

Characteristic features of striped muscle

(A) Composed of *unbranched* parallel fibres (compare with cardiac muscle which is branched)

(B) Numerous cross-striations visible

(C) Peripheral nuclei in fibres

Functions

(A) Voluntary body movements

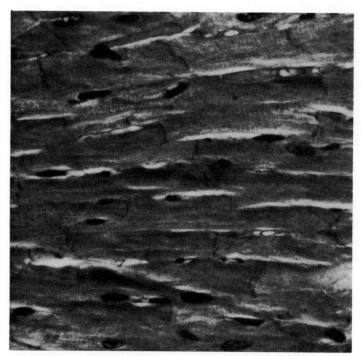

Fig. 6.2.(a)   Cardiac muscle (rat), L.S., high power. ×700

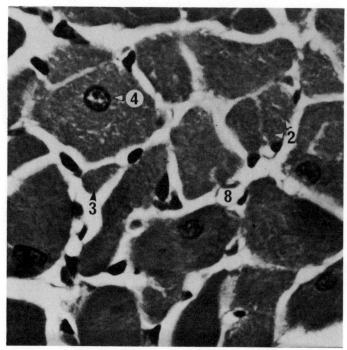

Fig. 6.2.(b)   Cardiac muscle (rat), T.S., high power showing a
              branch (3) of one of the fibres, central nuclei (4),
              myofibrils (2) and capillaries (8). ×1300

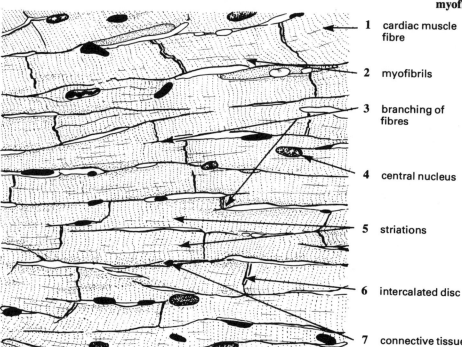

1   cardiac muscle
    fibre

2   myofibrils

3   branching of
    fibres

4   central nucleus

5   striations

6   intercalated disc

7   connective tissue
    between fibres

Fig. 6.2.(c)   Drawing of (a) showing characteristic branching (3)
              of fibres, central nuclei (4), striations (5) and
              intercalated discs (6)

*Characteristic features of cardiac
muscle*

(A)   Composed of numerous
branched fibres (compare with striped
muscle)

(B)   Cross-striations visible

(C)   Central nuclei in fibres
(compare with striped muscle)

(D)   Intercalated discs between ends
of fibres

Functions

(A)   Rapid rhythmical and
involuntary contraction of wall of
heart

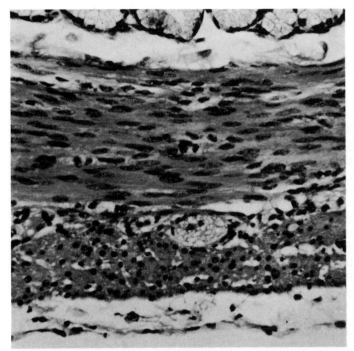

Fig. 6.3.(a) Smooth muscle (rat, gut), medium power, bundles of fibres cut in various planes. ×320

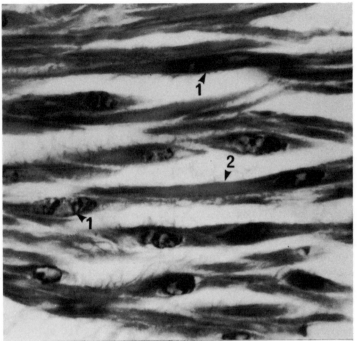

Fig. 6.3.(b) Smooth muscle (e.g. cow, gut), high power of longitudinally sectioned fibres (2) which have become artificially separated during preparation. Note elongate nuclei (1). ×1270

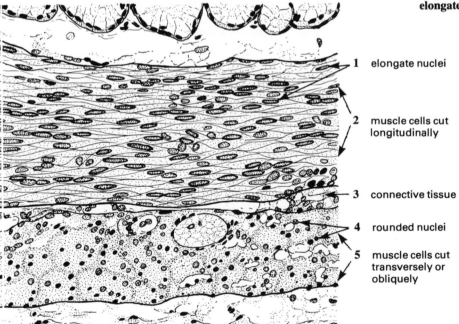

Fig. 6.3.(c) Drawing of (a). Note elongate nuclei (1) where bundles in L.S. and rounded nuclei (4) in T.S. or oblique sections

1 elongate nuclei

2 muscle cells cut longitudinally

3 connective tissue

4 rounded nuclei

5 muscle cells cut transversely or obliquely

6 muscularis externa of gut

Characteristic features of smooth muscle

(A) Composed of unbranched parallel fibres arranged in bundles

(B) No striations present

(C) Nuclei elongate in longitudinal sections

Functions

(A) Responsible for involuntary movements, e.g. peristalsis of intestine and uterine contractions

7 Blood and Vascular System

7.1 BLOOD

Blood (plus lymph), together with connective tissue proper, cartilage and bone, is a type of connective tissue which, as such, arises from the embryonic *mesenchyme* (*see* Chapter 5). Blood is a red liquid which functions to transport food, waste products, oxygen, hormones, etc., around the body and thus maintain homeostasis (= equilibrium) of the internal environment. It forms about 7 per cent of the body weight and is composed of the plasma or interstitial substance (= 55 per cent of the volume of blood), which contains many salts, enzymes, hormones, etc., in solution, and the cellular components (= 45 per cent of the volume of blood). These include the red blood corpuscles (= *erythrocytes*), the white blood cells (= *leucocytes*) and the blood platelets (= *thrombocytes*). The best way of studying these cells is in a thin blood film which has been stained with a special stain such as Giemsa or Wright's stain (*see* Giemsa technique, section 2.1.7(i)).

7.1.1 Erythrocytes

These (Fig. 7.1) are by far the most common cellular element in the blood, and in humans and rats there are 4–6.5 million/cu. mm (4–6.5 million per μl) and 9–9.5 million/cu. mm (9–9.5 million per μl) of blood, respectively. In mammals, they *lose their nuclei* during the last stage of development in the bone marrow and appear in blood smears as biconcave discs with very little internal structure visible. In fresh blood viewed under the microscope, erythrocytes sometimes stick together to form stacks or *rouleaux* and, if the plasma becomes hypertonic due to evaporation, they may appear star-like or *crenated*. The erythrocytes are composed of approximately two-thirds water and one-third solids, of which *haemoglobin* is the main constituent. In the lungs, haemoglobin combines easily with oxygen to form oxyhaemoglobin which is then transported around the body and gives up its oxygen to the tissues in areas of low oxygen tension.

7.1.2 Leucocytes

These (Fig. 7.1) are easily identified in blood smears after staining with Giemsa or Wright's stain as their nuclei stain a bright red/purple colour. They are much less common than erythrocytes with 5000–10000/cu.mm (5000–10000 per μl) in man and 6000–18000/cu. mm (6000–18000 per μl) in the rat. Each of the various types of leucocytes has a specific shape to the nucleus and characteristic staining of the cytoplasmic inclusions. Thus neutrophils, eosinophils, basophils, lymphocytes and monocytes can be identified free in the blood (Fig. 7.1). Neutrophils, eosinophils and basophils are sometimes collectively referred to as polymorphonuclear leucocytes or polymorphs because of their possession of a polymorphous (lobed) nucleus. Fixed macrophages (called histiocytes and developed by growth of monocytes) and mast cells are present in various other connective tissues such as the areolar tissue (*see* section 5.3.1). Frequently, the white cells are classified into two broad categories: *granular leucocytes* (= neutrophils, eosinophils and basophils) and *agranular leucocytes* (= lymphocytes and monocytes). The figures in this chapter indicate the structural characteristics and functions of each of the types of leucocytes.

7.1.3 Blood platelets

These (Fig. 7.1j) are also *anucleate* and appear as groups of small darkly staining rods or discs between the other cell types. There are approximately 300000/cu. mm (300000 per μl) in man and 800000/cu. mm (800000 per μl) in the rat. They represent cytoplasmic fragments produced by the disintegration of giant cells, the *megakaryocytes* (Fig. 7.3), which are found in the bone marrow. Disintegrating platelets function during blood clotting by releasing *thromboplastin* which is concerned in the formation of thrombin which together with *fibrinogen* (a plasma protein) forms the fibrin of the *blood clot*. They also agglutinate at the site of injury and help to plug the wound.

7.1.4 Bone marrow (= myeloid tissue)

The formation of the erythrocytes and the polymorphs (granular leucocytes) takes place in the *red bone marrow* (Fig. 7.3). In the foetus and newborn, all the bone marrow is red but as ageing occurs the red is partially converted to yellow (fatty, non-functional) bone marrow. In the adult, red bone marrow occurs mainly in the ribs, sternum, vertebrae, skull and proximal epiphyses of the femur and humerus. Red bone marrow together with the *lymphoid tissues* represent the only *haemopoietic* (= blood-cell forming) tissues in the body. The lymphoid tissue produces the lymphocytes and perhaps also the monocytes (= agranular leucocytes), although many believe that the latter arise in the bone marrow. The monocytes make their way to the various connective tissues and glands (e.g. lungs, spleen and liver) and subsequently mature and enlarge to form the fixed macrophages or histiocytes which filter out bacterial invaders. This sytem of fixed phagocytic macrophages forms the *reticulo–endothelial system* of the body. The reticuloendothelial cells of the spleen also ingest and destroy worn out erythrocytes.

7.2 VASCULAR SYSTEM

Oxygenated blood from the lungs passes back to the heart from which it is pumped to large arteries, small arteries, arterioles, capillaries (of the tissues and glands), venules, small veins, and finally to large veins which convey the deoxygenated blood back to the heart and thence to the lungs for reoxygenation. This system of blood vessels transporting the blood is the blood vascular system, and usually the arteries contain oxygenated blood and the veins deoxygenated blood.

7.2.1 Arteries

Three types of arteries are recognised:

(1) the large *elastic arteries,*
(2) the medium-sized *muscular arteries,* and
(3) the small *arterioles.*

The walls of these arteries consist of three basic layers (Fig. 7.2):

(1) *tunica intima* (= innermost layer) composed of an *endothelial* lining (= squamous epithelium of mesodermal origin) plus some connective tissue below it,
(2) *tunica media* (= middle layer) containing smooth muscle and connective tissue, and
(3) *tunica adventitia* (= outer layer) composed mainly of connective tissue.

The boundary between the tunica intima and tunica media is marked by the *internal elastic membrane,* while between the tunica media and the tunica adventitia the thinner *external elastic membrane* is found. The different types of arteries show some considerable variations in the structure of the three basic layers and in the thickness of the elastic membranes. Thus, the tunica media of large elastic arteries (e.g. *aorta*) is composed largely of elastic tissue while that of muscular arteries contains mainly smooth muscle cells. Muscular arteries are the most common type of artery and are characterised by a very well developed internal elastic membrane (*see* Fig. 7.2). The elastic nature of the walls of the arteries converts the intermittent flow of blood from the heart into a continuous flow throughout the body. Their elastic recoil acts as a secondary pump to advance the blood. The contraction and relaxation of the smooth muscle in the tunica media of the arterioles also greatly influence the blood pressure.

7.2.2 Veins

Veins have much larger lumens and thinner walls than arteries (Fig. 7.2) and the blood pressure in them is low. Various types of veins are also recognised, including small, medium and large. Their walls also have the same three layers as the arteries, i.e. tunica intima, tunica media and tunica adventitia, although the extent of these layers is often indistinct. The smooth muscle and elastic tissue in these layers are also poorly developed. Movement of blood in the veins is usually maintained by compression of their thin walls during contraction by the surrounding muscles of the body. Flow of the blood to the heart is ensured by valves in the veins which prevent the backflow of the blood.

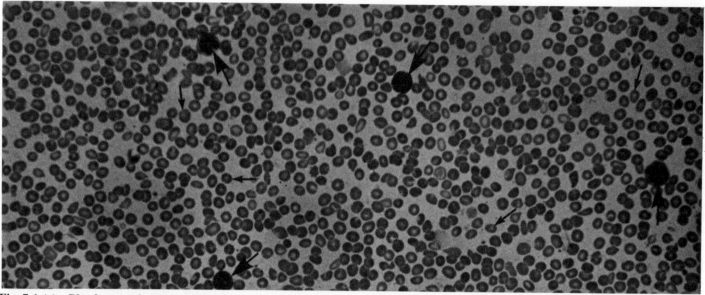

Fig. 7.1.(a)   Blood smear (human), low power, showing numerous non-nucleated erythrocytes (small arrows) and a few nucleated leucocytes (large arrows). Giemsa stain. ×430

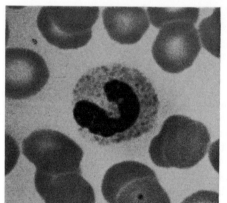

Characteristics

Horseshoe- or doughnut-shaped, nonsegmented nucleus, cytoplasmic granules

Functions

Rapidly matures, nucleus becomes segmented, and then the cell phagocytoses and kills bacteria

Fig. 7.1.(b)   Immature polymorph or band cell. ×2000

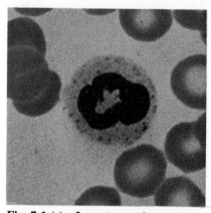

Characteristics

Horseshoe- or doughnut-shaped, nonsegmented nucleus, cytoplasmic granules

Functions

Rapidly matures, nucleus becomes segmented, and then the cell phagocytoses and kills bacteria

Fig. 7.1.(c)   Immature polymorph or band cell. ×2000

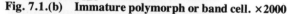

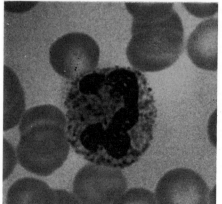

Characteristics

Multilobed nucleus, more cytoplasm than nucleus, cytoplasm contains many fine granules (lysosomes); 65–75% of leucocytes

Functions

Phagocytoses and kills bacteria

Fig. 7.1.(d)   Mature polymorph (neutrophil type). ×2000

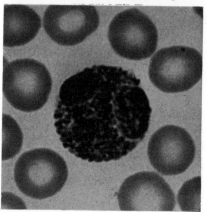

Characteristics

Nucleus often has two lobes, large amount of cytoplasm which contains characteristic large, orange, granules; 2–5% of leucocytes

Functions

Involved in allergic reactions together with mast cells, also rejection of parasites and phagocytosis

Fig. 7.1.(e)   Mature polymorph (eosinophil type). ×2000

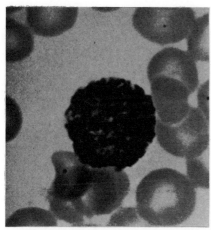

Characteristics

Same size as neutrophils; like mast cells, nuclear detail often masked by dark-staining granules; about 0.5% of leucocytes

Functions

Probably allergic reactions together with eosinophils and mast cells

Fig. 7.1.(f)   Mature polymorph (basophil type). ×2000

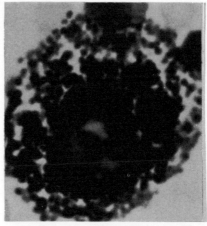

Characteristics

Very like large basophils with numerous dark-staining granules; and, as with macrophages, mainly confined to connective tissues and not free in blood

Functions

Contains many pharmacologically active substances involved in allergic and inflammatory reactions

Fig. 7.1.(g)   Mast cell (from peritoneal cavity of rat). ×2000

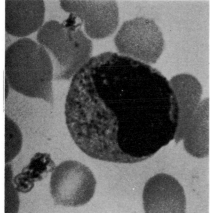

Characteristics

Large cells with a non-lobed, kidney-shaped nucleus, medium amount cytoplasm with fine granules (lysosomes); 3–8% leucocytes

Functions

Phagocytoses and kills bacteria, may enlarge into macrophages which assist lymphocytes in antibody production

Fig. 7.1.(h)   Monocyte. ×2000

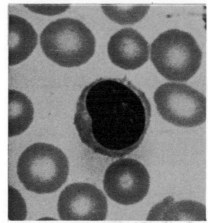

Characteristics

Vary in size, often smallest leucocyte type, composed mainly of round nucleus with thin rim of agranular cytoplasm; 20–30% of leucocytes

Functions

Complex immune reactions, e.g. antibody production and graft rejection

Fig. 7.1.(i)   Lymphocyte. ×2000

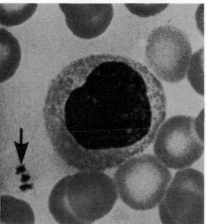

Characteristics

Such cells are very common. This one appears intermediate between a lymphocyte (large round nucleus, no cytoplasmic granules) and a monocyte (large cell, medium amount of cytoplasm). Note platelets (arrow)

Fig. 7.1.(j)   Intermediate cell type. ×2000

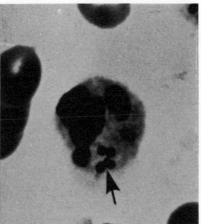

Phagocytosis

This is the ingestion by cells of foreign bodies, e.g. bacteria. The bacterium is recognised and binds to the leucocyte membrane, pseudopods form and draw it into the cytoplasm within a vacuole (= phagosome) and then lysosomes fuse with the phagosome and discharge enzymes, etc., to kill and degrade the microbe

Fig. 7.1.(k)   Phagocytic cell (neutrophil) containing ingested bacteria (arrow). ×2000

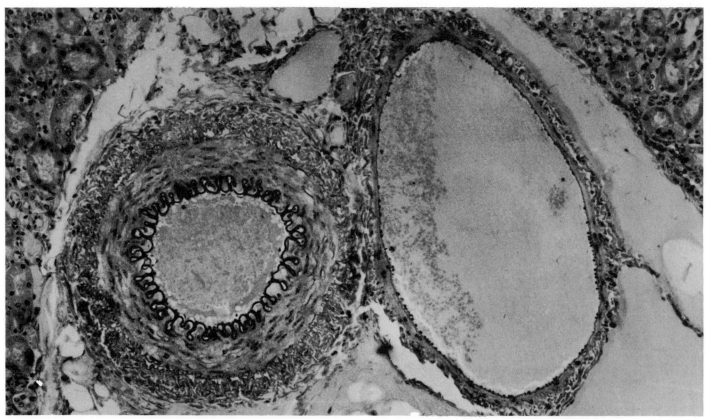

Fig. 7.2.(a)   Artery and vein (rabbit) in T.S. for comparative purposes. Note large lumen and thin wall of vein and smaller lumen and
                thicker wall of artery. ×200.

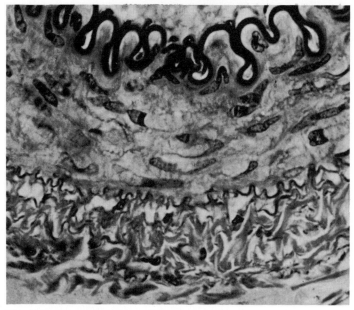

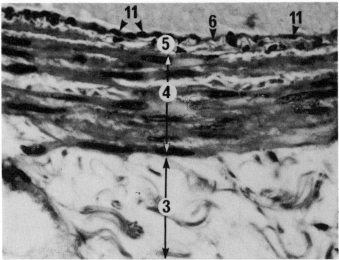

Fig. 7.2.(b)   Artery wall (rabbit), high power showing details of
                layers in the thick wall. ×700

Fig. 7.2.(c)   Vein wall (mammal), high power showing details of
                layers in the thin wall. Note indistinct tunica intima
                (5) composed of endothelial cells (11) lining lumen,
                and thin internal elastic membrane (6). The tunica
                media (4) is also thin and a tunica adventitia (3) is
                present. ×600

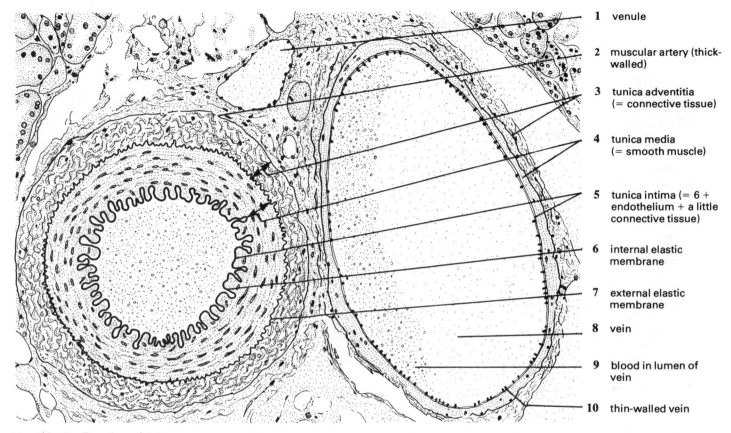

1   venule

2   muscular artery (thick-walled)

3   tunica adventitia (= connective tissue)

4   tunica media (= smooth muscle)

5   tunica intima (= 6 + endothelium + a little connective tissue)

6   internal elastic membrane

7   external elastic membrane

8   vein

9   blood in lumen of vein

10   thin-walled vein

Fig. 7.2.(d) Drawing of (a)

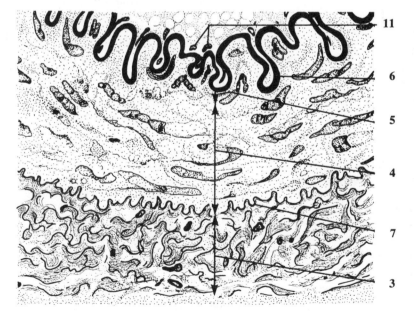

Fig. 7.2.(e) Drawing of (b). Note endothelial cells (11) lining lumen

Arteries versus veins

	Feature	Artery	Vein
(A)	lumen	restricted	large
(B)	wall	thick	thin
(C)	internal elastic membrane	thick	thin or absent
(D)	tunica media	thick	thin
(E)	tunica adventitia	thick	may be thick
(F)	external elastic membrane	present	absent

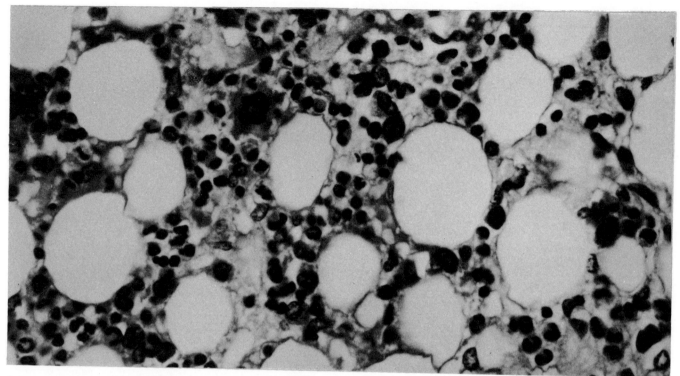

Fig. 7.3.(a)   Red bone marrow (from rat, longbone), low power, T.S. ×800

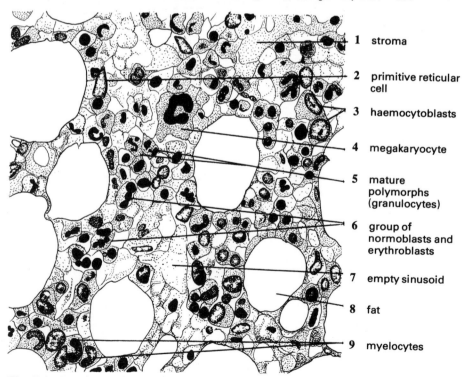

1 stroma

2 primitive reticular
   cell

3 haemocytoblasts

4 megakaryocyte

5 mature
   polymorphs
   (granulocytes)

6 group of
   normoblasts and
   erythroblasts

7 empty sinusoid

8 fat

9 myelocytes

Fig. 7.3. (b)   Drawing of part of (a)

Characteristic features of bone marrow

(A)   Sponge-like tissue with a fibrous stroma containing fat cells and many free cells of varied form

(B)   Giant megakaryocytes with lobed (polymorphous) nuclei usually present

(C)   No nervous, muscular, glandular or epithelial elements present

(D)   In sections of *whole* bone (not above) many sinusoids apparent

Functions

(A)   Haemopoiesis— formation of blood cells— which occurs chiefly in red and not yellow (fatty) bone marrow as follows: *primitive reticular cells ➝ haemocytoblasts* ➝ which form:

(i)   megakaryocytes ➝ platelets

(ii)   erythroblasts ➝ normoblasts ➝ erythrocytes

(iii)   myelocytes ➝ metamyelocytes ➝ three sorts of polymorphs, i.e. neutrophils, eosinophils and basophils (*see* blood, section 7.1.2)

8 Respiratory System

Inspired air passes into the nose/mouth→pharynx→larynx→trachea→bronchi→bronchioles and thence into the lungs for respiratory exchanges to take place (*see* Fig. 8.1). Such exchanges are essential in order to eliminate the waste carbon dioxide produced by metabolism and to take in oxygen which is utilised by the cells during energy production, synthesis, secretion, excretion, etc. Gaseous exchange occurs only in the *lungs;* the other parts of the respiratory system, sometimes collectively called the *respiratory passages,* serve to conduct air to and from these organs. Many of the passages are lined by *pseudostratified columnar epithelium* containing *goblet cells* (Fig. 8.2) which produce mucus to moisten the air and to trap foreign particles from the air before they reach the lungs. The surfaces of these cells are ciliated and move the mucus-entrapped particles towards the mouth and nose. The walls of the *trachea* and *bronchi* also contain *cartilaginous supports* which serve to keep the airways open (Figs 8.2 and 8.3). The goblet cells and cartilaginous supports gradually disappear as the bronchi pass into the lung tissue to become less than 1 mm in diameter and form the *bronchioles*. Bronchioles are lined by simple *ciliated columnar epithelium,* and as these pass from terminal to respiratory bronchioles the cilia are gradually lost and the epithelium becomes discontinuous (Fig. 8.4). The *respiratory bronchioles* open into the *alveolar ducts,* from which large numbers of air sacs or *alveoli* arise, and these greatly increase the surface area of the lungs for gaseous interchange. The alveoli occupy the bulk of the lung, and their thin *squamous epithelial walls* overlie a network of pulmonary capillaries (Fig. 8.3) which facilitates rapid gaseous exchange. *Deoxygenated blood* is brought to the alveoli via the *pulmonary arteries* and *oxygenated blood* is transported back to the heart via the *pulmonary veins*. The alveolar walls also contain elastic tissue, which allows distension and contraction of the lungs, but which can only be observed with special stains.

The *respiratory passages* have other functions apart from respiratory exchanges. The nasal or olfactory mucosa contains the *olfactory glands* which together with the appropriate neurones impart the *sense of smell,* while the larynx is also modified for the *production of sound*.

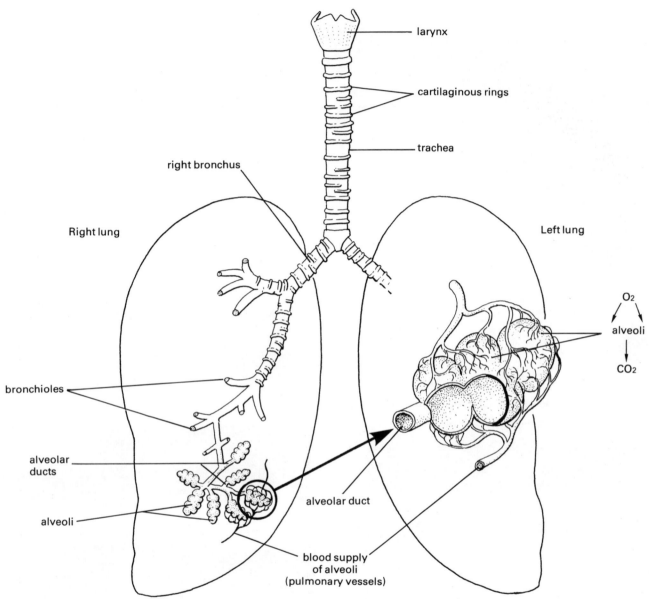

larynx

cartilaginous rings

trachea

right bronchus

Right lung

Left lung

O_2

alveoli

CO_2

bronchioles

alveolar
ducts

alveolar duct

alveoli

blood supply
of alveoli
(pulmonary vessels)

Fig. 8.1.   Parts of the respiratory system

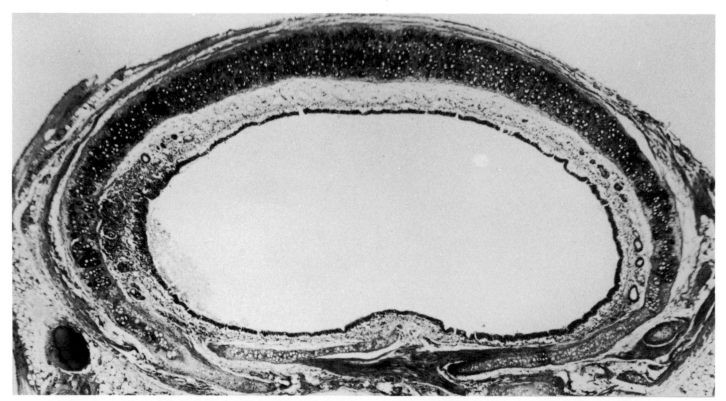

Fig. 8.2.(a)   Trachea (rat), low power T.S., Alcian Blue and haematoxylin stained. ×35

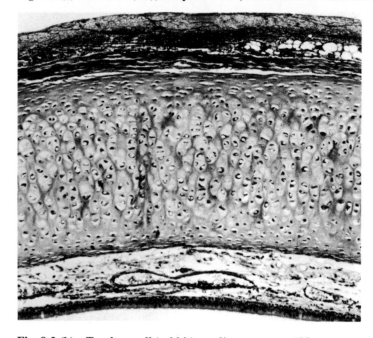

Fig. 8.2.(b)   Trachea wall (rabbit), medium power. ×105

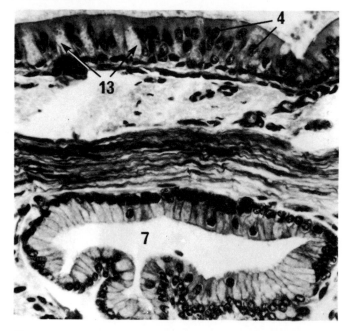

Fig. 8.2.(c)   Ciliated pseudostratified columnar epithelium (4) and ducts of glands (7) of trachea (sheep), high power. Note goblet cells (13). ×380

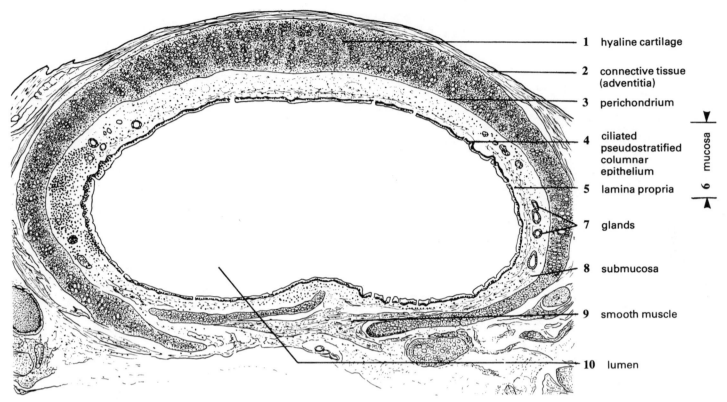

1 hyaline cartilage

2 connective tissue (adventitia)

3 perichondrium

4 ciliated pseudostratified columnar epithelium

5 lamina propria

6 mucosa

7 glands

8 submucosa

9 smooth muscle

10 lumen

Fig. 8.2.(d)   Drawing of (a)

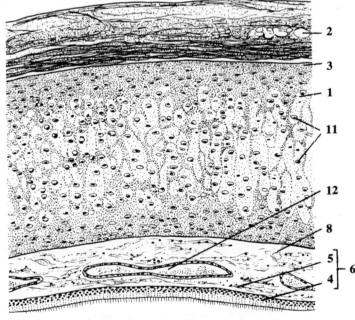

2

3

1

11

12

8

5

4

6

Characteristic features of trachea

(A)   Tubular, like gut; but in contrast has no villi, crypts or muscularis externa

(B)   Ciliated pseudostratified columnar epithelium present

(C)   C-shaped hyaline cartilaginous supports most characteristic feature

Functions

(A)   Passage for air to lungs

(B)   Warms, moistens and cleans air — mucus from glands traps dust and cilia waft it to nose and mouth

Fig. 8.2.(e)   Drawing of (b). Cartilage-secreting cells (chondrocytes) (11), blood vessels (12).
N.B. **No glands evident in this micrograph**

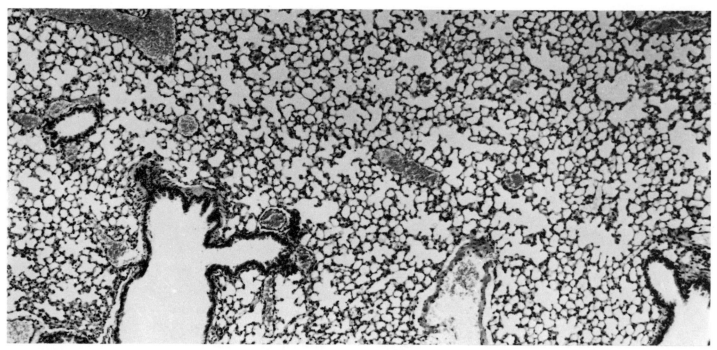

Fig. 8.3.(a)   Lung (mouse), low power, section. ×40

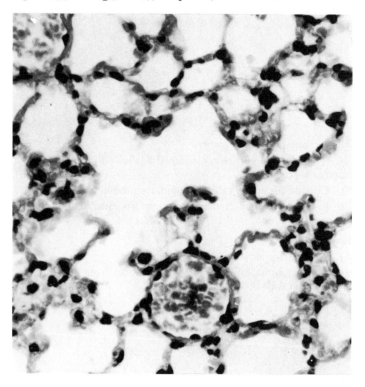

Fig. 8.3.(b)   Lung (mouse), high power, showing details of
alveoli. ×320

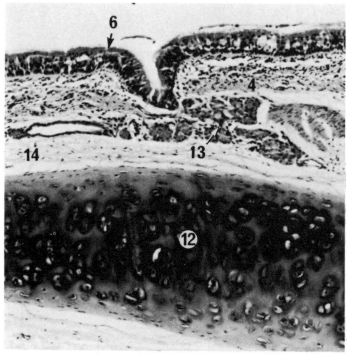

Fig. 8.3.(c)   Bronchus wall (baboon), medium power. Note
characteristic cartilaginous support (12) and
glandular tissue (13). Ciliated columnar epithelium
(6), connective tissue (14), smooth muscle (4). ×125

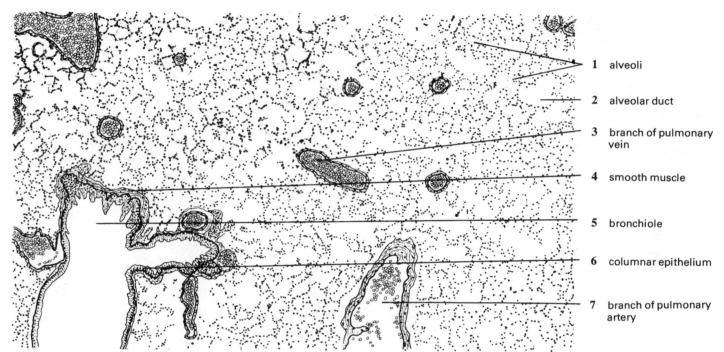

1 alveoli

2 alveolar duct

3 branch of pulmonary vein

4 smooth muscle

5 bronchiole

6 columnar epithelium

7 branch of pulmonary artery

Fig. 8.3.(d) Drawing of (a)

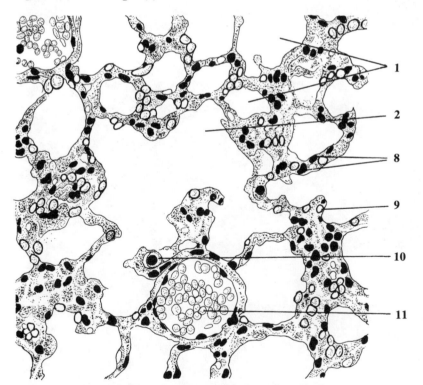

1

2

8

9

10

11

Fig. 8.3.(e) Drawing of (b) showing details of alveoli (1), nuclei (8) in endothelial and connective tissue cells of alveolar wall (9). Note also phagocytes (10) and capillary (11)

Characteristic features of lung

(A) Empty-looking, lace-like tissue composed of numerous thin-walled sacs

(B) Ramified by many tubular organs (= bronchi, bronchioles, ducts and blood vessels)

(C) Little skeletal (only cartilage) and glandular tissue present, and found only in wall of bronchi

(D) Muscular tissue scarce and confined to walls of respiratory tubes (bronchi and bronchioles)

Functions

(A) Respiratory interchange of gases across the walls of alveoli which are richly supplied with blood capillaries

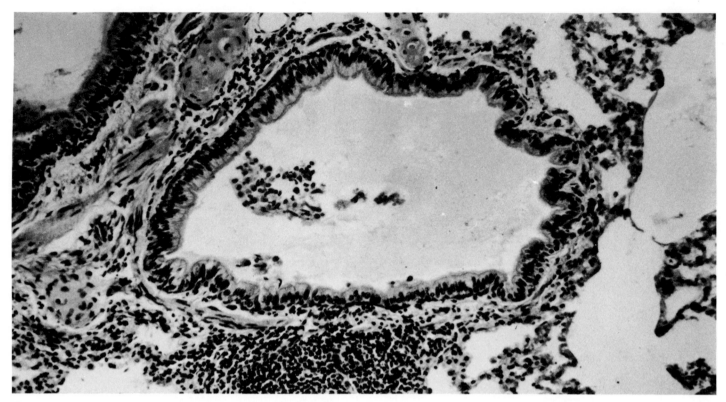

Fig. 8.4.(a)   Lung (rabbit), medium power of bronchiole. ×230

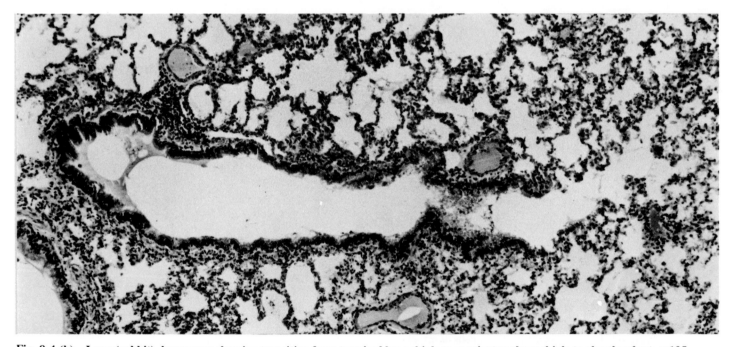

Fig. 8.4.(b)   Lung (rabbit), low power showing transition from terminal bronchiole to respiratory bronchiole to alveolar duct. ×105

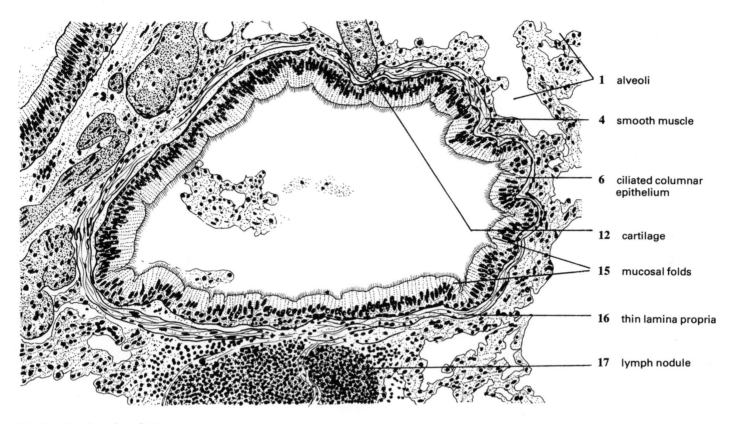

1 alveoli

4 smooth muscle

6 ciliated columnar epithelium

12 cartilage

15 mucosal folds

16 thin lamina propria

17 lymph nodule

Fig. 8.4.(c)   Drawing of (a)

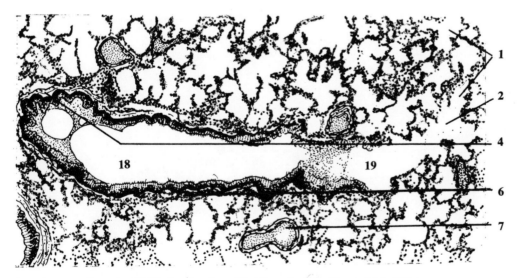

1

2

18   19

4

6

7

Passage of air

Air passes into nose → pharynx → larynx → trachea → bronchus → bronchiole → terminal bronchiole → respiratory bronchiole → alveolar duct → alveoli → alveolar wall → blood

Fig. 8.4.(d)   Drawing of (b) showing transition from terminal bronchiole (18) to respiratory bronchiole (19). Alveolar duct (2), pulmonary artery (7). ×75

9 Integumentary System (Skin)

Skin is one of the largest organs of the body and has many functions, including the protection of the body from the adverse effects of the environment. It also receives stimuli from the outside world.

9.1 STRUCTURE

Skin (Figs 9.1 and 9.2) basically consists of two layers, the *epidermis* and the *dermis*, which rest on a layer of connective tissue (often fat) called the *hypodermis*. The epidermis is a layer of *stratified squamous epithelium* containing keratinised outer layers (= *stratum corneum*) which are constantly being shed from the body and replaced by cells derived from the mitotic activity of the innermost epidermal layer, the *stratum germinativum*. Between the stratum germinativum and the stratum corneum are the *stratum spinosum* (= prickle cell layer; many desmosomes present between adjacent cells give them a prickly appearance) and the *stratum granulosum*. As the cells pass from the stratum germinativum to the stratum corneum, they become progressively flattened, accumulate keratohyalin granules (hence stratum granulosum) and become keratinised. Various modifications of the epidermis include the sweat glands, hair follicles, sebaceous glands and nails. Melanin, which protects the body from excessive ultraviolet light, is also synthesised in the epidermis.

The dermis consists mainly of *fibrous connective tissue* and contains the sweat glands, hair follicles, hair roots, arrector pili (= smooth muscle which elevates the hairs), sebaceous glands, a layer of striated muscles, the *panniculus carnosus* (which allows movements of the skin in many mammals), blood vessels, lymphatic vessels and two types of nerve endings, the *Meissner's* (located just below epidermis) and *Pacinian* (located deep in dermis) corpuscles (Fig. 9.2) which register touch and pressure, respectively. Pacinian corpuscles are also found in other organs of the body, e.g. pancreas.

9.2 CLASSIFICATION

Although the basic structure of skin (described above) is the same in different parts of the body, there is some considerable structural variation from one region to another. As a result of this variation, skin is sometimes classified as *thick* or *hairless,* and *thin* or *hairy*. Thick or hairless skin (Fig. 9.2) is found on the palms of the hands and soles of the feet, whilst thin or hairy skin (Fig. 9.1) covers the rest of the body. Thick skin has a very thick epidermis and the stratum corneum is particularly well developed and protects against wear and tear. Thick skin also has numerous sweat glands and nerve endings but no hair follicles. The skin of some small mammals, such as the rat, is devoid of sweat glands since overheating is not the problem that it is in large mammals such as man.

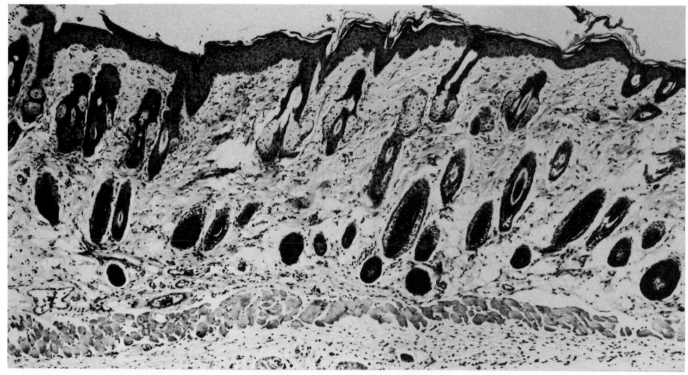

Fig. 9.1.(a)   Thin or hairy skin (mouse), low power section. ×80. *N.B.* **No sweat glands**

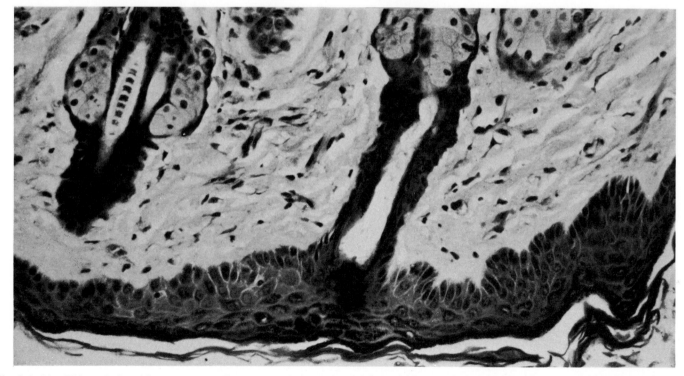

Fig. 9.1.(b)   Thin or hairy skin (mouse), medium power showing details of the epidermis, hair follicle and sebaceous glands. ×300

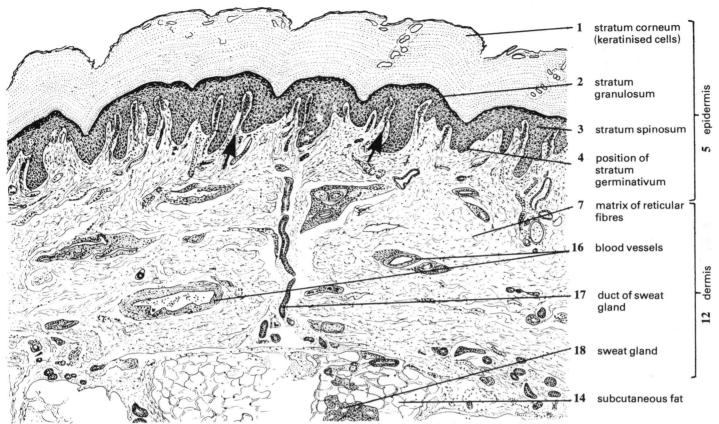

1 stratum corneum (keratinised cells)

2 stratum granulosum

3 stratum spinosum

4 position of stratum germinativum

5 epidermis

7 matrix of reticular fibres

16 blood vessels

17 duct of sweat gland

18 sweat gland

14 subcutaneous fat

12 dermis

Fig. 9.2.(d) Drawing of (a). Compare thickness of stratum corneum (1) with that of Fig. 9.1. Note Meissner's corpuscles (arrows)

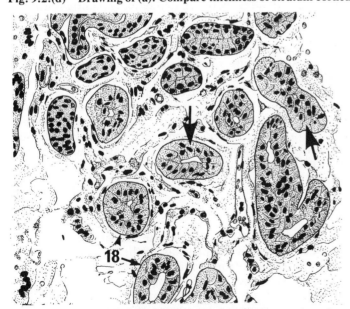

Fig. 9.2.(e) Drawing of (b), high power of secretory region of alveoli of sweat gland (18). Note columnar secretory cells (unlabelled arrows)

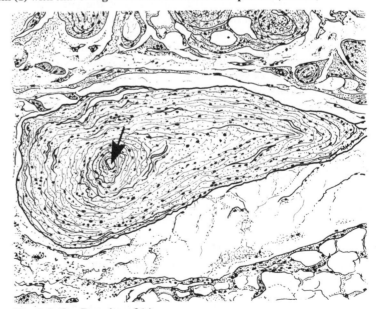

Fig. 9.2.(f) Drawing of (c)

10 Lymphoid Tissues*

Scattered throughout the body there are aggregations of large numbers of lymphocytes, and such foci form the lymphoid tissues. Lymphoid tissues usually stain extremely darkly with haematoxylin and eosin, since lymphocytes have very little cytoplasm and the cells thus mainly take up the nuclear stain (haematoxylin). The lymphoid tissues produce lymphocytes and plasma cells, and as such are termed haemopoietic (blood cell forming). The other main haemopoietic centres in the body are found in the bone marrow (see Fig. 7.3).

10.1 CLASSIFICATION AND STRUCTURE

10.1.1 Lymph nodules

Lymphoid tissues are found in the form of *small non-encapsulated nodules* (Figs 10.1 and 10.2) in the gut and respiratory system. In the gut, they are frequently concentrated in the ileum to form the *Peyer's patches* (Fig. 10.1), in the *appendix* of the large intestine (Fig. 10.2) and form the *tonsils* around the beginning of the digestive system. Each nodule may develop a light-staining *germinal centre* of dividing cells which form lymphoblasts and young lymphocytes. These lymphatic nodules are concentrated in regions such as the gut which are likely to be invaded by micro-organisms.

10.1.2 Lymph nodes

Frequently, *large encapsulated masses* of lymphoid tissue are found associated with the lymphatic system. These structures are termed *lymph nodes* (Fig. 10.3) and often occur in groups along the lymphatic vessels. They are particularly common in the groins, axillae and mesenteries, where they are composed of groups of lymph nodules with well defined, usually lighter-staining, *germinal centres*. The fibrous *capsule* forms *trabeculae* of connec-

tive tissue which penetrate the lymph node between the nodules. Most of the nodules are confined to the outer region of the lymph node, which is termed the *cortex,* while the inner region, or *medulla,* is composed of *cords* of dense lymphoid tissue. An indentation called the *hilus* makes the lymph node kidney-shaped and may assist in its identification.

Lymph nodes serve to filter the lymph and remove foreign bodies and cell debris. Below the capsule, between the nodules and in the medulla are *sinuses* or *sinusoids* which contain elements of the *reticulo-endothelial system* (fixed phagocytes) which ingest particulate matter and so clear the lymph. Lymph is carried to the nodes via afferent lymphatic vessels and movement through the nodes is maintained by the muscular movement of the body.

10.1.3 Thymus

The thymus (Fig. 10.4) is very similar to a lymph node in structure, and each of its two lobes is composed of a number of *lobules* with lighter-staining centres which resemble the nodules in the cortex of a lymph node. However, these central regions are *not germinal* but just contain fewer lymphocytes and lymphoblasts than the outer darker-staining regions and they are characterised by the presence of Hassall's corpuscles composed of concentric layers of flattened epithelial cells.

The thymus, like the lymph node, has a fibrous *capsule* and trabeculae, but, in contrast, the organ as a whole does *not* have a *central medulla* composed of cords of dense lymphoid tissue. The thymus declines in size and becomes fatty with increasing age.

10.1.4 Spleen

The spleen (Fig. 10.5) lies in the upper part of the abdomen directly in the pathway of the circulating blood which it *filters* and from which it removes worn-out red blood cells. It is, like the liver, composed of red, soft tissue and microscopically consists of small lymph nodules (= *white pulp*) surrounded by masses of reticular fibres and

*See Fig. 3.1 for location of various organs.

red blood cells (= *red pulp*). In haematoxylin and eosin stained sections, however, the white pulp stains darkly (= lymphocytes and lymphoblasts which take up the nuclear stain), while the red pulp stains lighter (= mainly red cells which have no nuclei and take up the cytoplasmic stain, i.e. the eosin). Although *germinal centres* may develop in the white pulp and the organ is *encapsulated* and has connective tissue trabeculae, it can often be distinguished from the lymph node and thymus by the dark staining of the centres of the lymph nodules (white pulp).

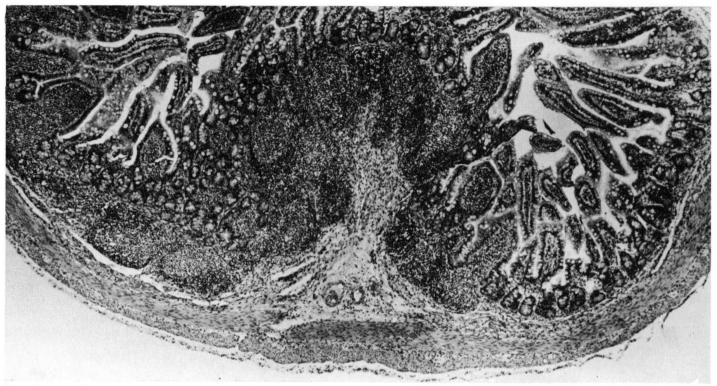

Fig. 10.1.(a)   Ileum (rat), low power showing lymph nodules. T.S. ×50

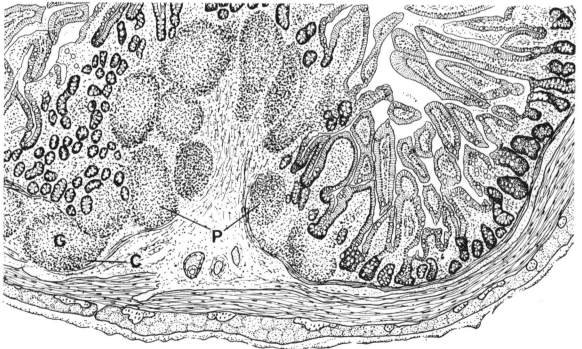

For detailed labelling *see* ileum (Fig. 11.13). The lamina propria of the small intestine contains numerous lymph nodules which in the ileum form groups called Peyer's patches (P). Each nodule may be subdivided into a germinal centre (G) and a cortex (C). Peyer's patches are visible to the naked eye as thickened white regions on the intestinal wall opposite the point of attachment of the mesentery

Fig. 10.1.(b)   Drawing of right-hand side of (a)

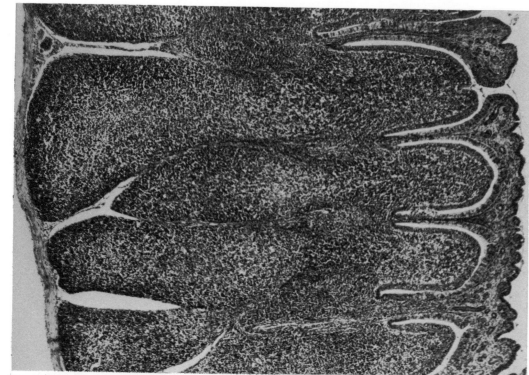

Fig. 10.2.(a)   Appendix (rabbit), low power T.S. ×50

Characteristic features of appendix

(A)   The four basic gut layers are present

(B)   Numerous lymph nodules

(C)   Few goblet cells present

(D)   Muscularis mucosae poorly developed

(E)   Submucosa sometimes obscured by lymph nodules

(F)   Muscularis externa thin

Functions

Unknown, but may play some role in development of antibody synthesising tissue

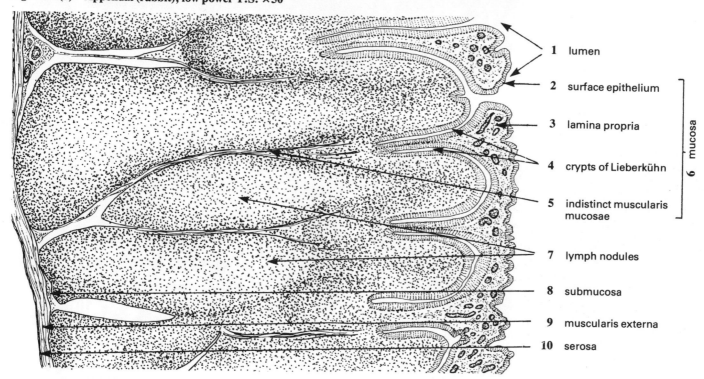

1   lumen

2   surface epithelium

3   lamina propria

4   crypts of Lieberkühn

5   indistinct muscularis mucosae

6   mucosa

7   lymph nodules

8   submucosa

9   muscularis externa

10   serosa

Fig. 10.2.(b)   Drawing of (a)

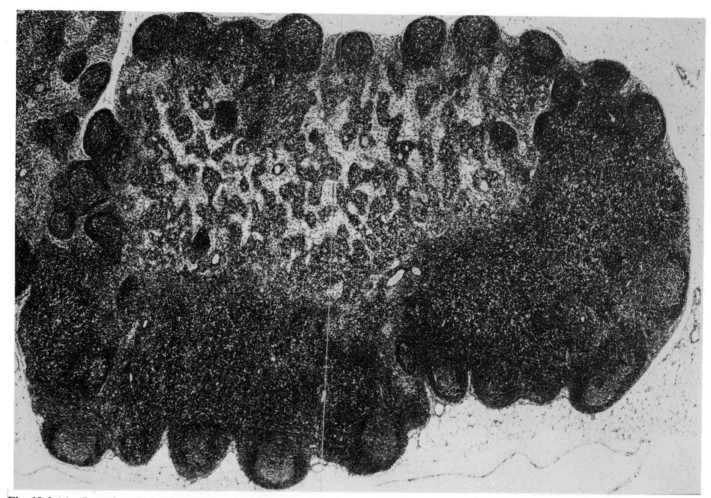

Fig. 10.3.(a)   **Lymph node (rabbit), low power. ×40**

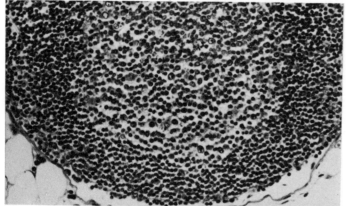

Fig. 10.3.(b)   **Lymph nodule (rabbit) from (a), medium power. Note outer region of closely packed small lymphocytes, central germinal centre of loosely packed larger lymphocytes and outer cortical sinus containing reticular cells. × 250**

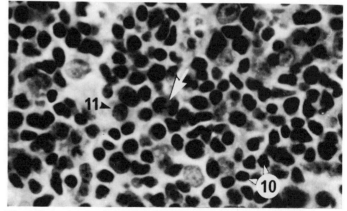

Fig. 10.3.(c)   **Germinal centre of lymph nodule (rabbit) from (a), high power. Note variation in size of lymphocytes from small (10) darkly staining to large (11) lighter staining cells. Mitotic cells are also present (unlabelled arrow). × 970**

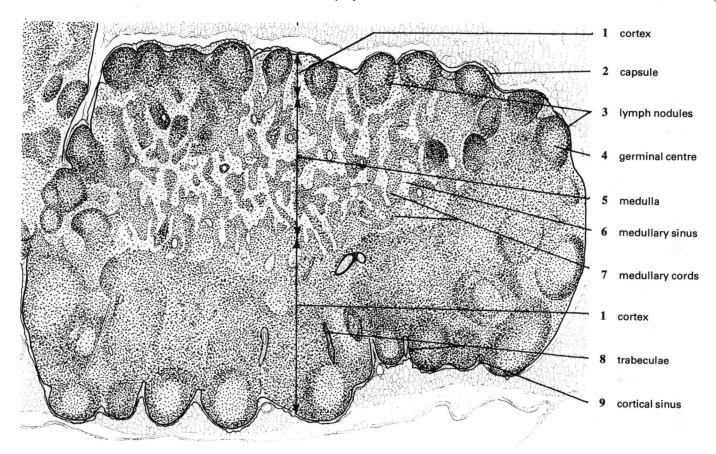

1	cortex
2	capsule
3	lymph nodules
4	germinal centre
5	medulla
6	medullary sinus
7	medullary cords
1	cortex
8	trabeculae
9	cortical sinus

Fig. 10.3.(d)   Drawing of (a). ×33

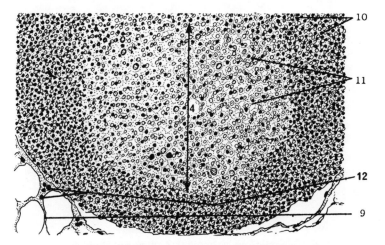

**Fig. 10.3.(e)   Drawing of (b). Note outer region of closely packed
small lymphocytes (10), central germinal centre (4)
of loosely packed larger lymphocytes (11) and
outer cortical sinus (9) containing reticular cells (12)**

Characteristic features of lymph node

(A)   Solid, darkly staining, often kidney-shaped, organ
divided into a cortex and medulla and surrounded by a
connective tissue capsule

(B)   Cortex contains numerous lymph nodules separated by
trabeculae and with lightly staining germinal centres containing
mitotic cells

(C)   Medulla composed of typical medullary cords which
distinguish lymph nodes from other lymphoid tissues (i.e.
spleen and thymus)

Functions

(A)   Filters lymph, and reticular cells (= phagocytes) remove
foreign particles

(B)   Some of ingested particles are presented to lymphocytes
which are stimulated to divide and mature to plasma cells
which produce antibodies

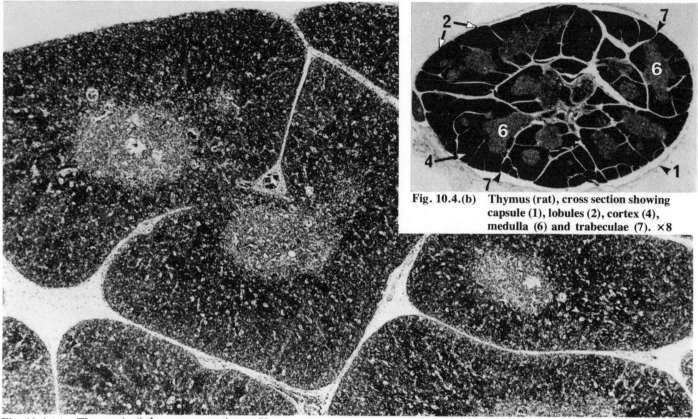

Fig. 10.4.(b)   Thymus (rat), cross section showing
                 capsule (1), lobules (2), cortex (4),
                 medulla (6) and trabeculae (7). ×8

Fig. 10.4.(a)   Thymus (rat), low-power section. ×50

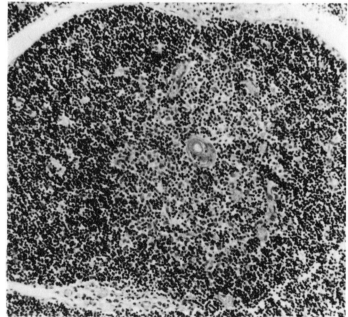

Fig. 10.4.(c)   Thymic lobule (human), medium-power section.
                 ×160

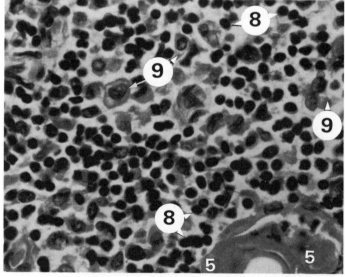

Fig. 10.4.(d)   Thymic lobule (human), high power showing two cell
                 types — darkly staining lymphocytes (8) in various
                 stages of development and lighter staining epithelial
                 reticular cells (9). Note also the characteristic
                 Hassall's corpuscle (5). ×700

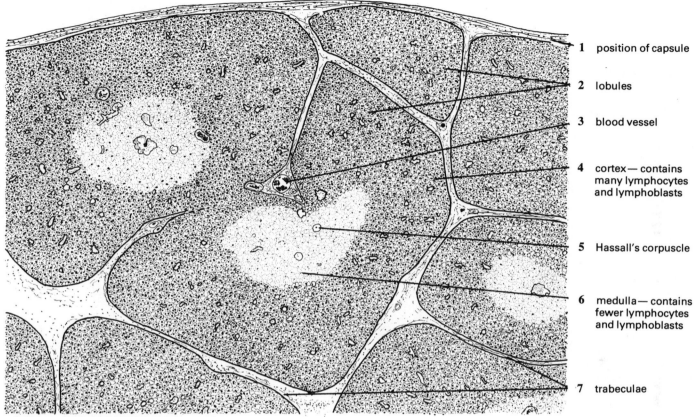

1 position of capsule

2 lobules

3 blood vessel

4 cortex — contains many lymphocytes and lymphoblasts

5 Hassall's corpuscle

6 medulla — contains fewer lymphocytes and lymphoblasts

7 trabeculae

Fig. 10.4.(e)   Drawing of (a)

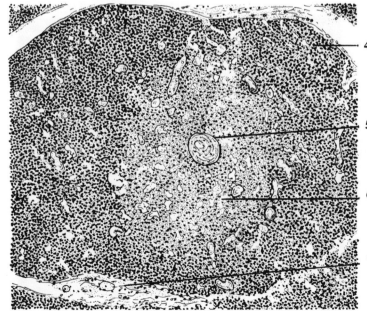

4

5

6

7

Fig. 10.4.(f)   Drawing of (c)

Characteristic features of thymus

(A)   Solid, darkly staining organ divided into lobules by inpushings (= trabeculae) from connective tissue capsule

(B)   Each lobule has a lightly staining centre (= medulla) which is surrounded by a darkly staining cortex (other way round in spleen)

(C)   Medulla contains one or more Hassall's corpuscles composed of concentric layers of flattened epithelial cells

(D)   Two cell types — lymphocytes (darkly staining) and epithelial reticular cells (lightly staining) present under high power

Functions

(A)   Produces T-lymphocytes which are responsible for cell-mediated immune responses, e.g. graft rejection

(B)   May also produce a thymic hormone (possibly in the epithelial reticular cells) which stimulates the production of the lymphocytes

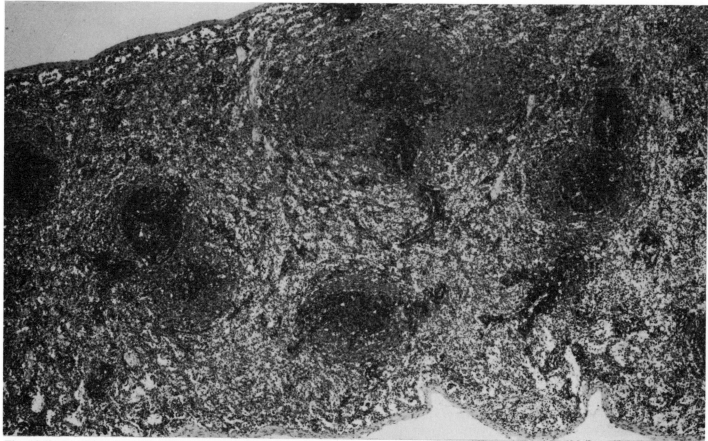

Fig. 10.5.(a)   Spleen (rat), low-power section. ×55

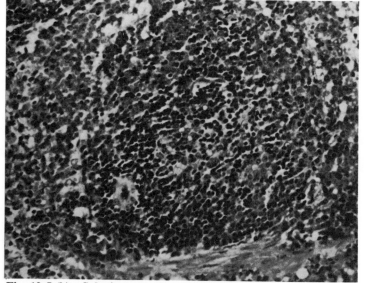

Fig. 10.5.(b)   Splenic corpuscle (rat), medium-power section. ×275

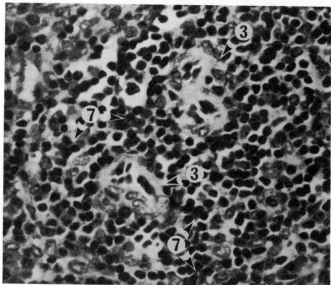

Fig. 10.5.(c)   Splenic corpuscle (rat), high-power section showing central arterioles (3) and lymphocytes and lymphoblasts (7) in germinal centre. ×500

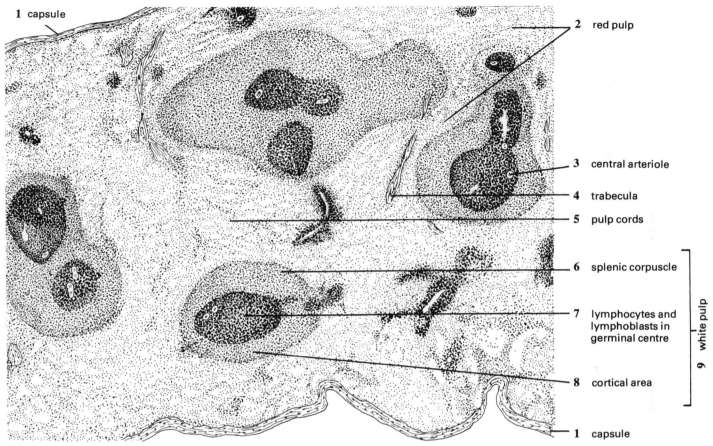

1 capsule
2 red pulp
3 central arteriole
4 trabecula
5 pulp cords
6 splenic corpuscle
7 lymphocytes and lymphoblasts in germinal centre
8 cortical area
9 white pulp
1 capsule

Fig. 10.5.(d)   Drawing of (a)

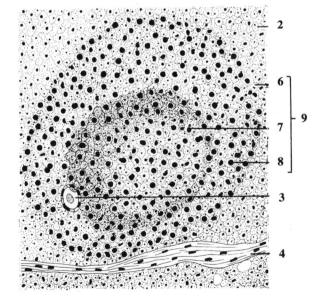

Fig. 10.5.(e)   Drawing of (b)

Characteristic features of spleen

(A)   Like thymus, has connective tissue capsule but, in contrast, not divided into distinct lobules

(B)   Infoldings of capsule = trabeculae

(C)   Darkly stained lymph nodules = white pulp

(D)   White pulp = lymphocytes (large nuclei)

(E)   Central arterioles in lymphatic nodules

(F)   Lighter-staining regions = red pulp

(G)   Red pulp contains erythrocytes

Functions

(A)   White pulp produces lymphocytes = germinal centres

(B)   Red pulp stores and filters blood, removes worn-out red cells

11 Digestive System and Associated Glands*

Food passes from the mouth ➝ pharynx ➝ digestive tube which consists of the oesophagus ➝ stomach ➝ small intestine (= duodenum, jejunum and ileum) ➝ large intestine (= caecum, appendix and colon) ➝ rectum ➝ anus. During its passage through the digestive system, the food is broken down by both mechanical and chemical means, nutrients are produced and absorbed into the body and indigestible substances are eliminated.

Every part of the digestive system has a key role to play in these processes. Thus, in the mouth, the *teeth* cut, tear and grind the food which is mixed with saliva synthesised in numerous *salivary glands* (parotid, submandibular = submaxillary, and sublingual) and which contains water, salts, mucus and sometimes enzymes that begin carbohydrate digestion. The *tongue* is highly muscular and rolls the food into a ball and passes it to the *pharynx* and thence

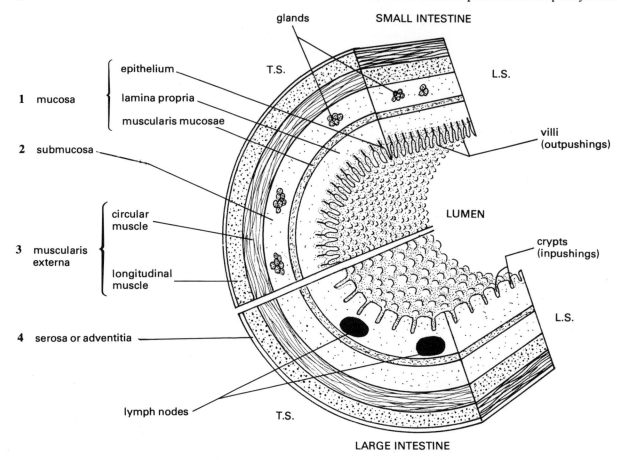

Fig. 11.1. Digestive tube showing the general arrangement of the four layers forming the wall

*See Fig. 3.1 for location of parts.

100

by the swallowing reflex to the first part of the digestive tube, the *oesophagus*. Micrographs of various parts of the digestive system are shown in Figs 11.2 to 11.20.

The wall of the *digestive tube* consists basically throughout its length of four layers (*see* Fig. 11.1):

(1) mucosa
    (a) epithelium
    (b) lamina propria
    (c) muscularis mucosae
(2) submucosa
(3) muscularis externa
    (a) circular muscle
    (b) longitudinal muscle
(4) serosa or adventitia

11.1 MUCOSA

This lines the lumen of the digestive tube and is composed of *three layers* as follows.

11.1.1 Epithelium

The epithelium, which borders the lumen, is in direct contact with the food. It is from the epithelium that the glands associated with the digestive system, such as the *crypts of Lieberkühn, Brunner's glands, oesophageal glands, liver* and *pancreas,* develop.

11.1.2 Lamina propria

The lamina propria is composed of connective tissue and supports the epithelium. It often contains blood and lymphatic vessels and lymph nodes. Products of digestion pass through the epithelium into the vessels in this layer.

11.1.3 Muscularis mucosae

The muscularis mucosae consists of smooth muscle fibres which move the mucosa. This layer is very obvious in the oesophagus (*see* Fig. 11.2), but may be difficult to see in the other parts of the digestive tube.

11.2 SUBMUCOSA

Like the lamina propria, this is composed of connective tissue but contains much larger blood vessels. Groups of nerve fibres (= *Meissner's plexus*) may also be present. In the oesophagus and duodenum, glands occur in the

submucosa. In the duodenum, they may be so well developed (= Brunner's glands) that they completely fill and mask this layer (*see* composite figure of digestive tube, Fig. 11.2).

11.3 MUSCULARIS EXTERNA

This is usually composed of *two layers of smooth muscle.* The fibres in the inner layer (i.e. nearest lumen) are arranged circularly and those in the outer layer longitudinally (*see* Fig. 11.1 above). These layers undergo peristaltic movements and propel the food along the digestive tube. These muscular movements are controlled by nerve fibres and ganglia called *Auerbach's plexus* (*see* Figs 11.11 and 11.14).

N.B. In any section of the gut, it is possible to determine the *plane of sectioning* by examining the arrangement of the muscle fibres in these two layers. If the fibres of the inner layer (the circular layer) are clearly seen to run around, i.e. encircle, the gut and the fibres of the outer layer (the longitudinal layer) are cut in cross section, then it is a transverse section (T.S.). The opposite applies in L.S., and both planes of sectioning together with the arrangement of the muscle fibres are illustrated in Fig. 11.1.

11.4 SEROSA

This is composed of a layer of *squamous epithelial cells* (mesothelium) and a little connective tissue, and is very thin and often difficult to see. This layer surrounds most of the digestive tube but is absent in places, e.g. around the oesophagus, which instead has a thick connective tissue layer called the *adventitia* (= tunica adventitia).

11.5 VARIATIONS IN STRUCTURE OF THE DIFFERENT REGIONS OF THE DIGESTIVE TUBE

Each region of the digestive tube (Fig. 11.2) has a specific function and this is reflected in the structure of the component layers, especially the mucosa. These differences are very obvious in the composite figure (Fig. 11.2) which shows four regions of the gut.

11.5.1 Oesophagus

This simply transports food to the stomach. The oesophagus is thus lined with *stratified squamous epithelium* to prevent wear and tear of the lining by the food, and has a thick muscular coat and a well developed muscularis mucosae to assist in movement of the food to the stomach.

11.5.2   Stomach

This receives the food from the oesophagus and begins chemical degradation. It has a very thick mucosa composed mainly of long *fundic* or *gastric glands* which produce hydrochloric acid and enzymes which begin the breakdown of proteins.

11.5.3   Small intestine

This is characterised by a mucosa thrown into numerous finger-like *villi* for food absorption and by invaginations at the base of the villi, the *crypts of Lieberkühn,* which make an important contribution to the production of the *intestinal juice.* The intestinal juice (= succus entericus) may contain a number of digestive enzymes, although there is evidence for the production of these elsewhere, for example in the absorptive cells.

In the duodenum only, the submucosa is characteristically filled by the *Brunner's glands,* which produce an alkaline secretion that neutralises the acidity of food from the stomach.

Note the difference in the structure between the villi (long finger-like outpushings) of the small intestine and the crypts (invaginations between angular portions of the gut wall) of the large intestine (Fig. 11.2).

11.5.4   Large intestine

The mucosa consists of numerous *tubular inpushings* or *crypts of Lieberkühn* (sometimes referred to as glands of Lieberkühn in the large intestine), which contain many goblet cells and produce mucus. No villi or digestive glands are present, and this region simply absorbs water from the food to form the faeces. Lymph nodules may be present in the lamina propria of most regions of the digestive tube but are especially developed in the large intestine.

11.6   ASSOCIATED GLANDS

These include the salivary glands (Fig. 11.4), liver (Figs 11.17 and 11.18), gall bladder (Fig. 11.19) and pancreas (Fig. 11.20). Apart from the liver, their structure is comparatively simple.

The pancreas and gall bladder both discharge their products into the duodenum, and these substances assist in digestion and absorption of foodstuffs. The pancreas also contains the islets of Langerhans, which have an endocrine function and secrete insulin and glucagon which lower and raise blood glucose levels, respectively. In haematoxylin and eosin stained preparations, all the component cells of the islets appear *identical,* but with special staining techniques, e.g. the chromium–haematoxylin–phloxine method (section 2.1.7(d)), it is possible to identify three kinds of granular cells: the *beta cells,* which are the most numerous (50–75% of cells), centrally located and responsible for *insulin* production; the *alpha cells,* which are usually peripherally located (form *ca* 20% of cells) and produce *glucagon;* and the *delta cells,* which are the least numerous (*ca* 5%) and may synthesise *somatostatin* which inhibits insulin and glucagon release (*see* Fig. 11.20).

The liver is the largest organ in the body, is enclosed within a thin connective tissue sheath and is composed of numerous epithelial cells (= the hepatic cells = hepatocytes) arranged into *lobules.* These lobules are hexagonal in section and may be clearly defined by a sheath of connective tissue (the *Glisson's capsule*), as in the pig, or more commonly are less well defined because of the reduction or absence of this sheath (Figs 11.17 and 11.18). The lobules can also be identified by the presence of the *portal areas* (*see* below) at their peripheries (Figs 11.17 and 11.18), and by the arrangement of the hepatocytes, which form cords of cells converging upon a blood vessel, the *central vein,* in the centre of each lobule. The structure (in section) is like that of a wheel, with the tyre representing the connective tissue sheath, the spokes equivalent to the cords of liver cells and the hub being the central vein.

A true understanding of liver structure and function, however, can only be obtained by considering the blood circulation in this organ. Blood *rich in digested foodstuffs* (amino acids, glucose, etc.) is transported from the intestine to the liver via the *portal vein,* while blood *rich in oxygen* enters the liver via the *hepatic artery.* Once in the liver, these two vessels divide repeatedly until each forms a small branch in the *portal areas* at the periphery of the lobules. From the portal areas, the portal vein and hepatic artery penetrate the lobules and send out numerous small branches to form the *sinusoids,* which are minute blood capillaries completely surrounding the liver cells and allowing for *metabolic exchanges* (e.g. glucose uptake from blood) between the blood and hepatocytes. The sinusoids eventually open into the *central vein* of each lobule and these unite to form the *hepatic vein* which joins the inferior vena cava that empties into the heart. The sinusoids also contain fixed phagocytes, the *Kupffer cells,*

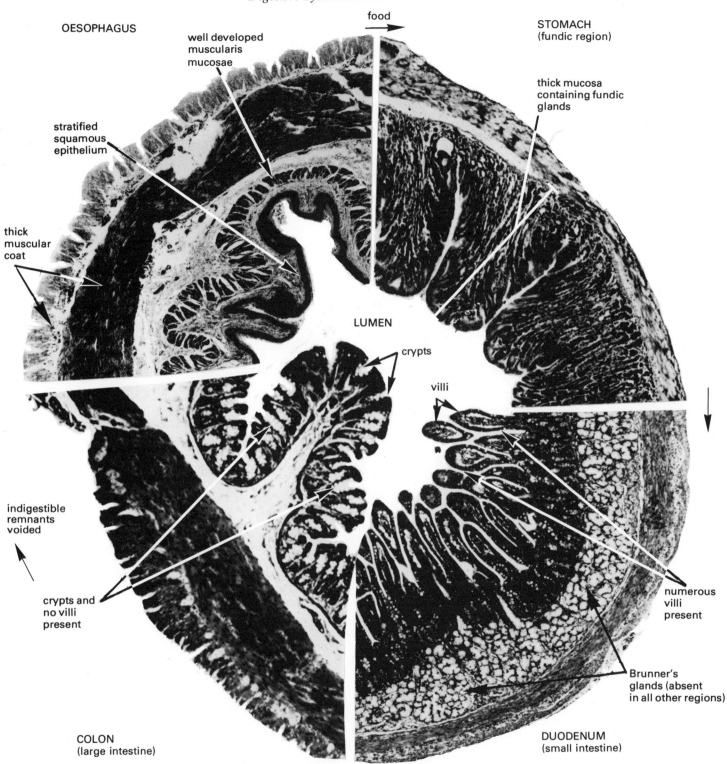

OESOPHAGUS

food

STOMACH
(fundic region)

well developed
muscularis
mucosae

thick mucosa
containing fundic
glands

stratified
squamous
epithelium

thick
muscular
coat

LUMEN

crypts

villi

indigestible
remnants
voided

crypts and
no villi
present

numerous
villi
present

Brunner's
glands (absent
in all other regions)

COLON
(large intestine)

DUODENUM
(small intestine)

Fig. 11.2. Composite micrograph of the digestive tube showing variations that exist between the different regions (*see* text for details).

which form part of the reticulo-endothelial system and clear the blood of foreign particles (e.g. bacteria). Between the hepatocytes, minute canals, the *bile canaliculi,* are also present (Fig. 11.18) and these serve to collect the bile produced by the hepatocytes. The bile caniculi unite to form the *bile ducts* of the portal area (Fig. 11.18), and these bile ducts eventually join into the *common hepatic duct* of the *gall bladder* which stores the bile until it is discharged into the duodenum.

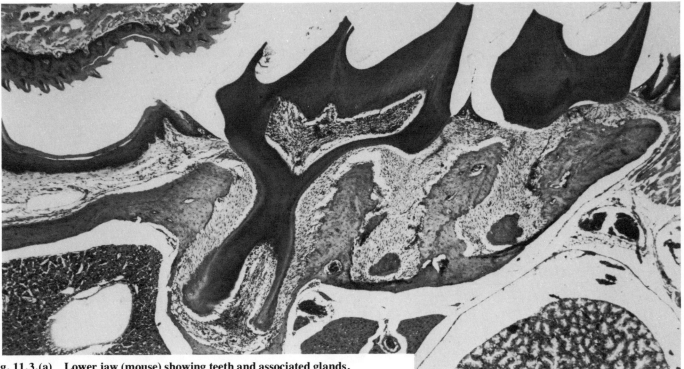

Fig. 11.3.(a) **Lower jaw (mouse) showing teeth and associated glands.**
Low power. ×50. *N.B.* Enamel dissolved away during
decalcification prior to sectioning

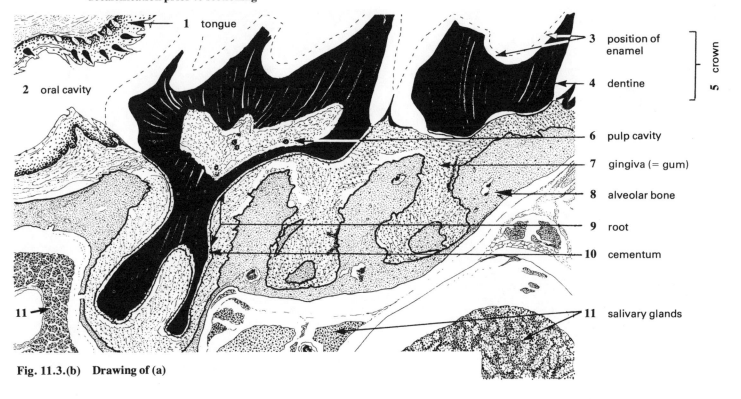

Fig. 11.3.(b) **Drawing of (a)**

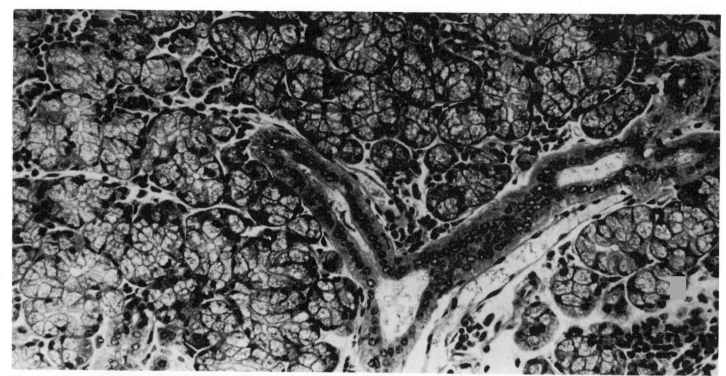

Fig. 11.4.(a)   Sublingual salivary gland (mainly mucous)(mouse), medium power. ×300. *N.B.* Striated and intercalated ducts infrequent, serous alveoli scarce

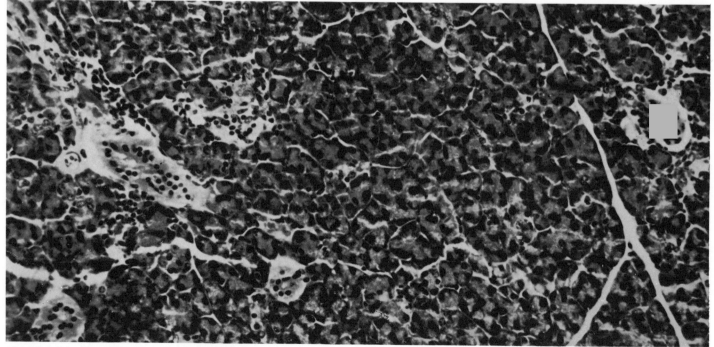

Fig. 11.4.(b)   Parotid salivary gland (mainly serous) (mouse), medium power. ×300. *N.B.* Composed purely of serous alveoli, striated ducts common and gland lobed

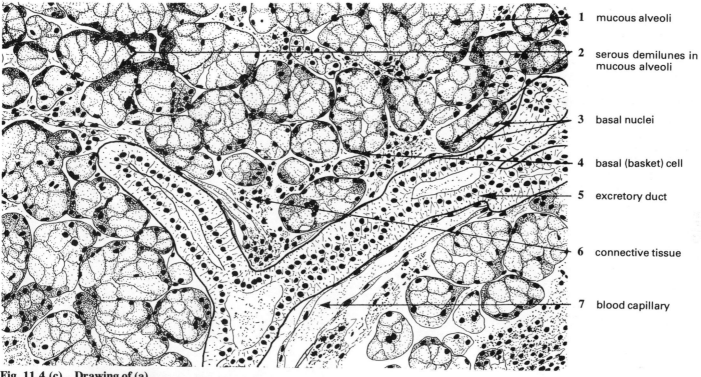

1 mucous alveoli

2 serous demilunes in mucous alveoli

3 basal nuclei

4 basal (basket) cell

5 excretory duct

6 connective tissue

7 blood capillary

Fig. 11.4.(c)   Drawing of (a)

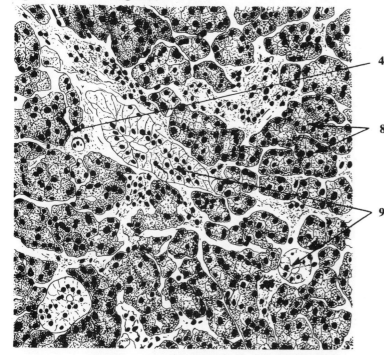

4

8

9

Fig. 11.4.(d)   Drawing of left-hand side of (b). *N.B.* **Composed purely of serous alveoli (8), striated ducts (9) common and gland lobed**

Characteristic features of salivary glands

(A)   Composed of masses of secretory alveoli

(B)   No complex muscle bands, villi or large blood vessels present

(C)   Mainly mucous glands (e.g. sublingual) stain lightly, mainly serous glands (e.g. parotid and submandibular) stain more intensely

(D)   Series of ducts drain alveoli

Functions

(A)   Production of mucus of saliva (in mucous alveoli), which prepares food for swallowing and digestion, cleans and moistens teeth and mouth

(B)   In some species, saliva contains enzymes (produced in serous alveoli) which begin carbohydrate digestion

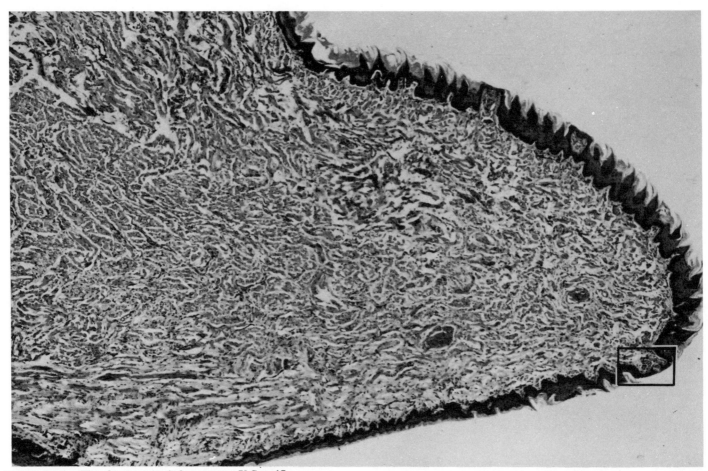

Fig. 11.5.(a)   Tip of tongue (rat), low power. V.S. ×45

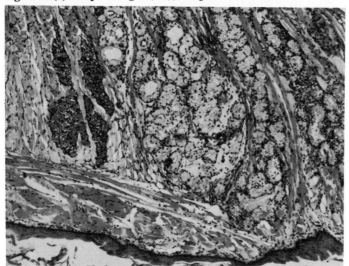

**Fig. 11.5.(b)   Tongue (rabbit), medium power showing serous
and mucous lingual glands. V.S. ×80**

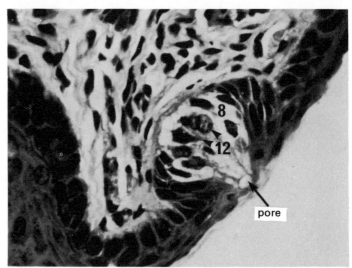

**Fig. 11.5.(c)   Taste bud (8) in fungiform papilla of tongue (rat),
high power(= boxed area in (a)). Note sensory
and supporting cells (12). ×640**

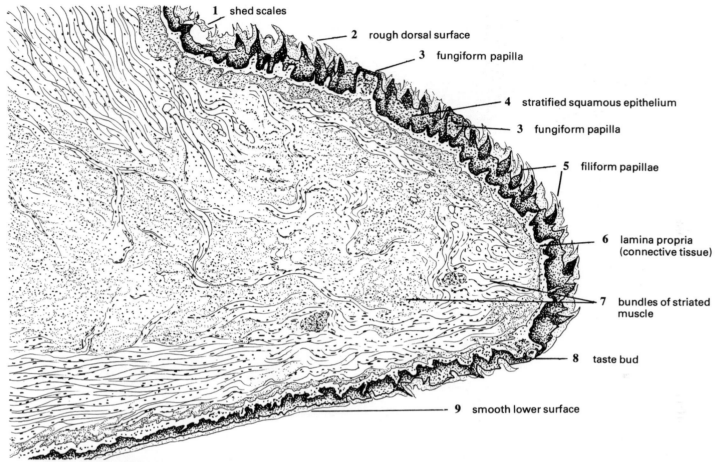

1 shed scales
2 rough dorsal surface
3 fungiform papilla
4 stratified squamous epithelium
3 fungiform papilla
5 filiform papillae
6 lamina propria (connective tissue)
7 bundles of striated muscle
8 taste bud
9 smooth lower surface

Fig. 11.5.(d)   Drawing of (a)

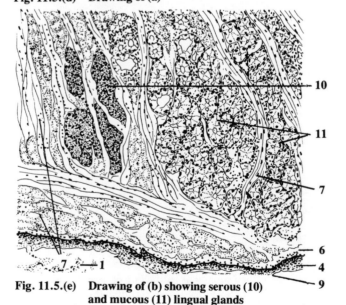

10
11
7
6
7   1
4
9

Fig. 11.5.(e)   Drawing of (b) showing serous (10) and mucous (11) lingual glands

Characteristic features of tongue

(A)   Typical shape

(B)   Stratified squamous epithelium present

(C)   Numerous dorsal projections (= papillae), ventral surface (underside) smooth

(D)   Numerous bundles of striated muscle fibres

(E)   Taste buds present in fungiform and vallate papillae (latter found only in posterior part of tongue), but absent from filiform papillae

Functions

(A)   Taste

(B)   Lapping of fluids

(C)   Formation of food ball

(D)   Assists swallowing

(E)   Communication

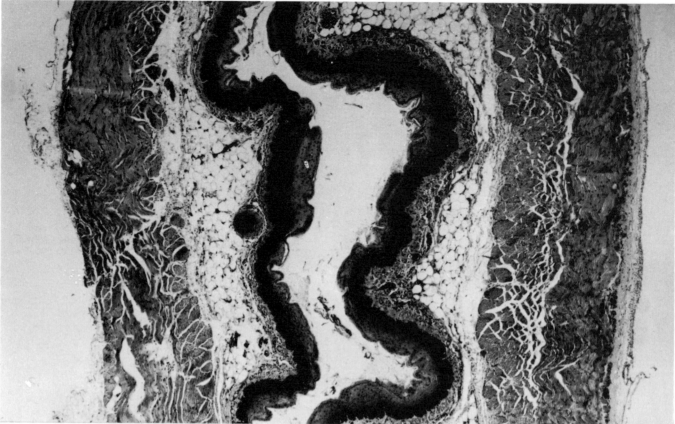

Fig. 11.6.(a)   Oesophagus (rabbit), low power. L.S. ×50

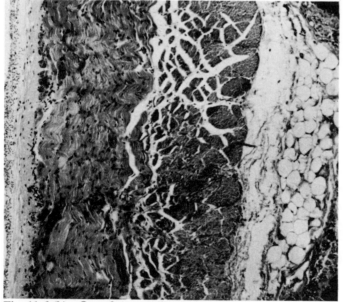

Fig. 11.6.(b)   Oesophagus wall (rabbit), medium power. ×80

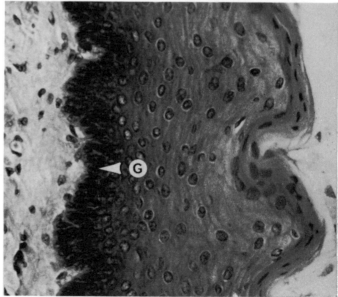

Fig. 11.6.(c)   Stratified squamous epithelium of oesophagus
                (rabbit) high power. Note germinal layer (G).
                ×280

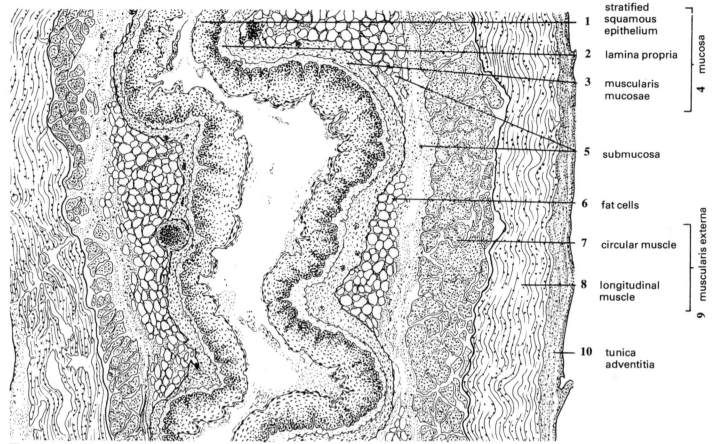

1 stratified squamous epithelium
2 lamina propria
3 muscularis mucosae
4 mucosa
5 submucosa
6 fat cells
7 circular muscle
8 longitudinal muscle
9 muscularis externa
10 tunica adventitia

Fig. 11.6.(d)   Drawing of (a)

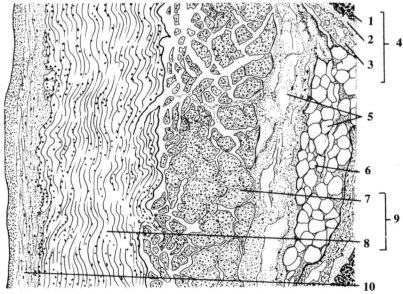

Fig. 11.6.(e)   Drawing of (b)

Characteristic features of oesophagus

(A)   No villi or crypts

(B)   Typical stratified squamous epithelium present

(C)   Few glands present except at lower end near stomach

(D)   Muscularis externa thick, two- or three-layered and may be, in contrast to much of gut, composed of striated muscle in upper parts

(E)   Covered by a thick layer of connective tissue (tunica adventitia)

Functions

(A)   Conveys food from pharynx to stomach by muscular movements (peristalsis)

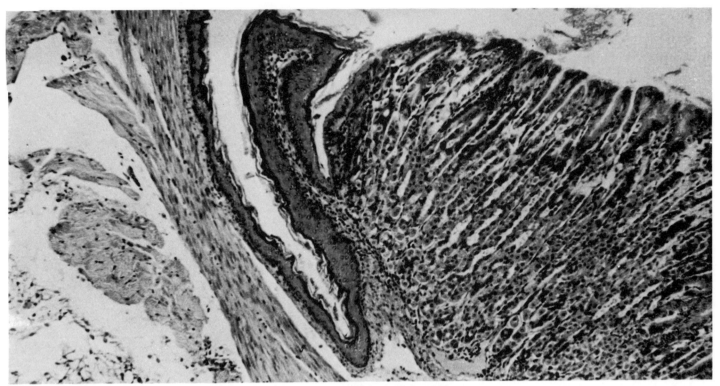

Fig. 11.7.(a) Oesophagus/stomach junction (= cardia) (mouse), low power T.S. ×100

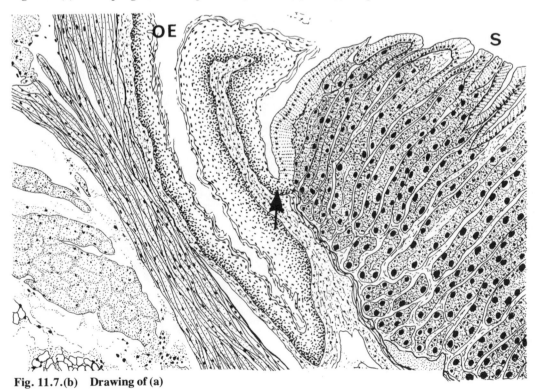

OE

S

Fig. 11.7.(b) Drawing of (a)

For detailed labelling, *see* oesophagus and stomach (Figs 11.6 and 11.8). Main feature to note is the replacement (unlabelled arrow) of the stratified squamous epithelium of the oesophagus (OE) by the simple columnar mucous epithelium of the stomach (S)

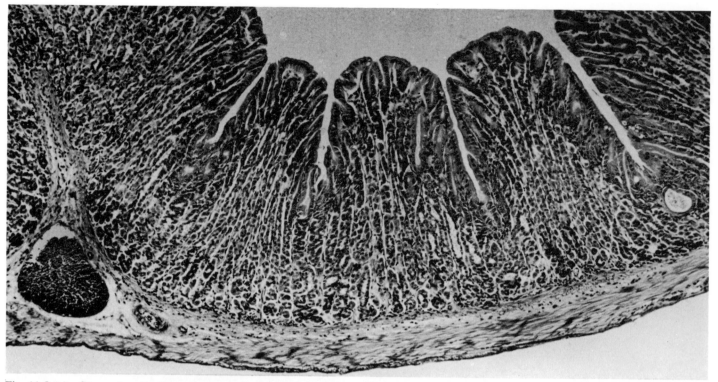

Fig. 11.8.(a)   Stomach — fundic region (mouse), lower power T.S. ×100

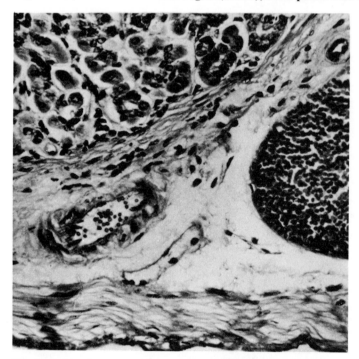

Fig. 11.8.(b)   Stomach wall (mouse), medium power showing parietal cells in fundic glands. T.S. ×300

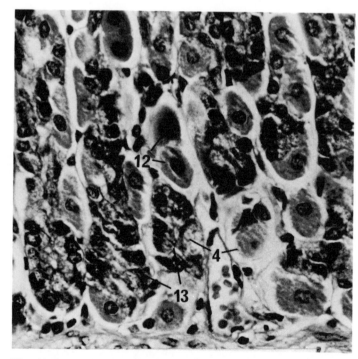

Fig. 11.8.(c)   Parietal (12) and chief (13) cells in fundic glands (4) of stomach (mouse), high power. ×600

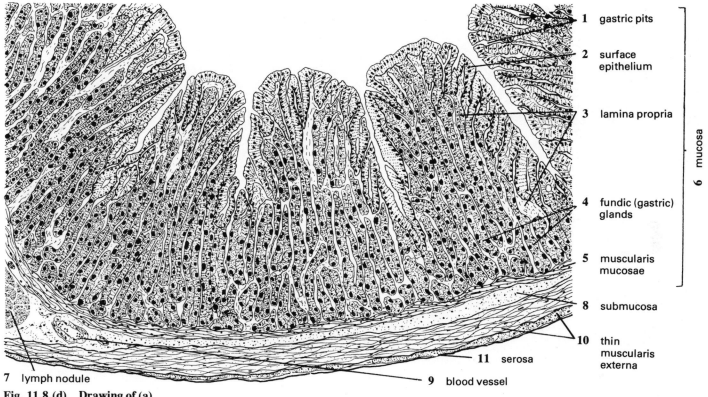

1 gastric pits
2 surface epithelium
3 lamina propria
4 fundic (gastric) glands
5 muscularis mucosae
6 mucosa
8 submucosa
10 thin muscularis externa
11 serosa
9 blood vessel
7 lymph nodule

Fig. 11.8.(d)   Drawing of (a)

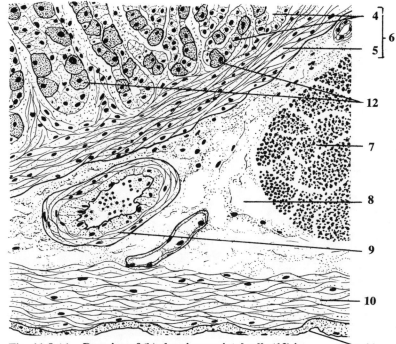

4
6
5
12
7
8
9
10
11

Fig. 11.8.(e)   Drawing of (b) showing parietal cells (12) in fundic glands (4)

Characteristic features of fundic region of stomach

(A)   Contains fundic (gastric) glands composed of parietal cells (produce HCl) and chief cells (produce enzymes)

(B)   Pits but no villi present (compare small intestine)

(C)   Often (but not in above section) has thick muscularis externa for mixing food

(D)   May be difficult to see the usual two outer muscle layers; a third oblique layer may also be present

Functions

(A)   Stores food from oesophagus

(B)   Digests food by action of muscles and gastric juice

(C)   Some water, glucose and alcohol absorbed

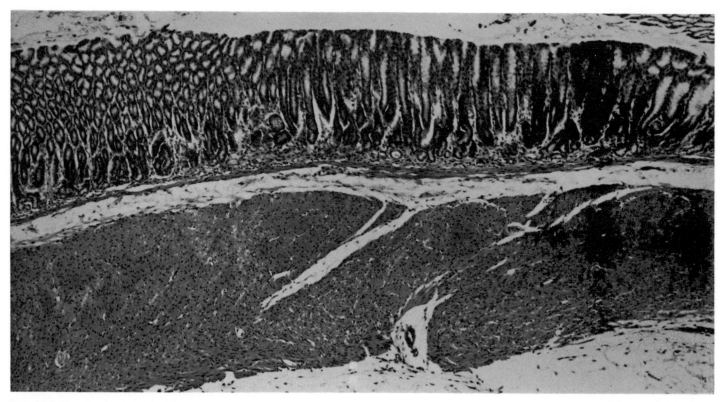

Fig. 11.9.(a)   Stomach — pyloric region (rat), low power. L.S. ×90

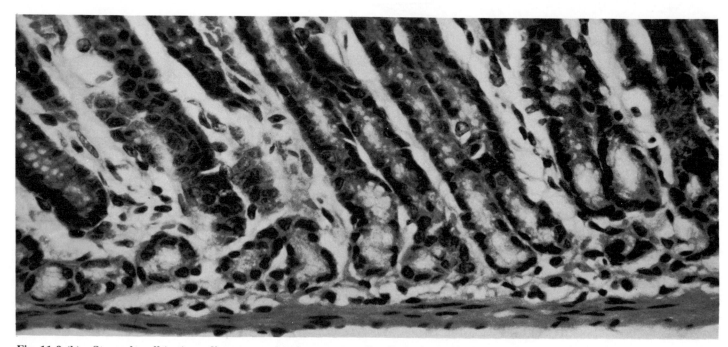

Fig. 11.9.(b)   Stomach wall (rat), medium power showing mucous cells of pyloric glands. L.S. ×400

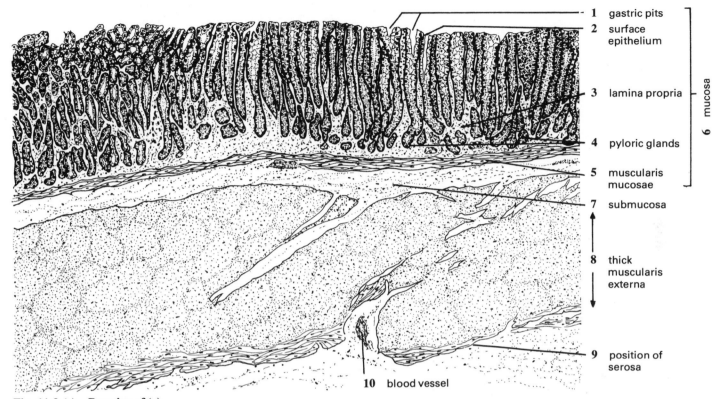

- **1** gastric pits
- **2** surface epithelium
- **3** lamina propria
- **4** pyloric glands
- **5** muscularis mucosae
- **6** mucosa
- **7** submucosa
- **8** thick muscularis externa
- **9** position of serosa
- **10** blood vessel

Fig. 11.9.(c)   Drawing of (a)

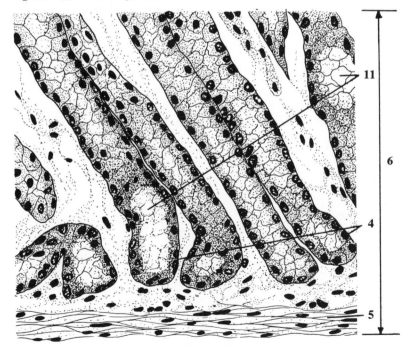

Fig. 11.9.(d)   Drawing of middle part of (b) showing mucous cells (11) of pyloric glands (4)

Characteristic features of pyloric region of stomach

(A)   Contains pyloric glands composed of one cell type = typical mucous cells (compare fundic glands of fundic region of the stomach which contain parietal and chief cells)

(B)   Pits but no villi present

(C)   Three muscle layers may be present (but are not clearly defined in (a)); circular layer (as seen in (a)) may be thick and form sphincter to control evacuation of stomach

(D)   Gastric pits deeper than in fundic region

Functions

(A)
(B)   } As for fundic region of stomach
(C)

(D)   Controls passage of food into duodenum by means of the pyloric sphincter

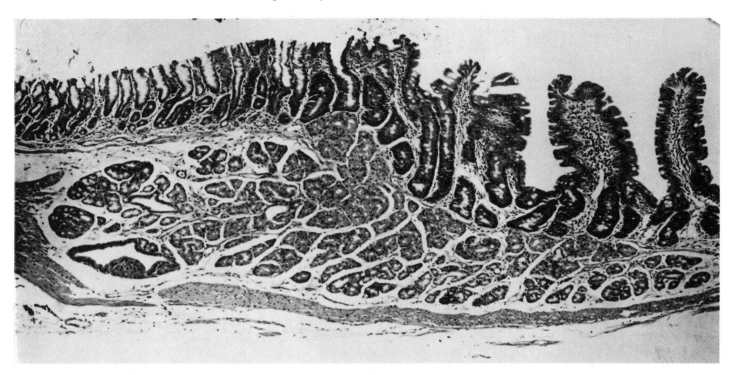

Fig. 11.10.(a)   Stomach/duodenum junction (rat), low power L.S. ×90

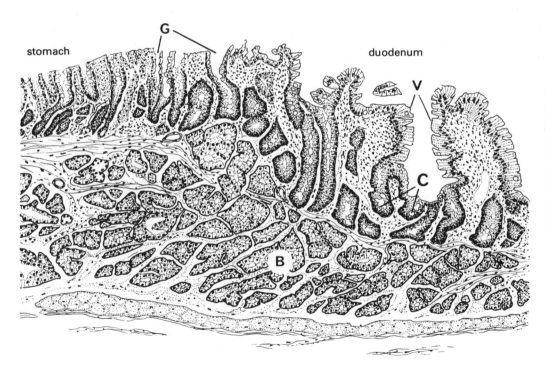

For detailed labelling, *see* pyloric region of the stomach and duodenum (Figs 11.9 and 11.11). This section illustrates clearly the transition from the gastric pits (G) of the pyloric region of the stomach to the comparatively large villi (V) and crypts of Lieberkühn (C) of the duodenum. The Brunner's glands (B) of the duodenum are well developed in the submucosa

Fig. 11.10.(b)   Drawing of (a)

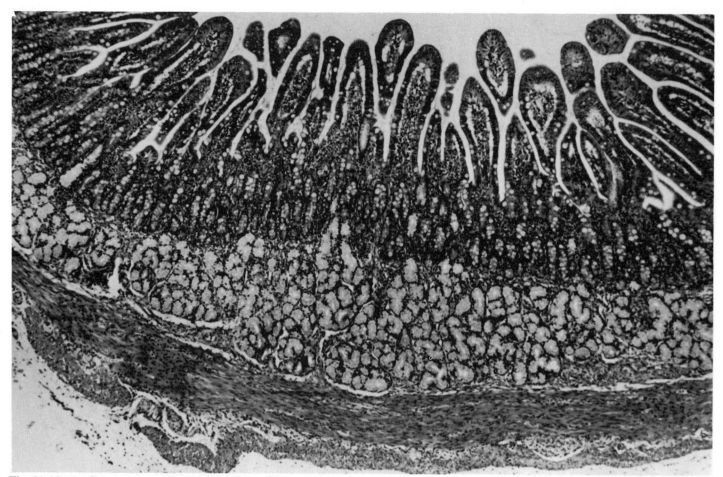

Fig. 11.11.(a)   Duodenum (rat), low power T.S. ×80

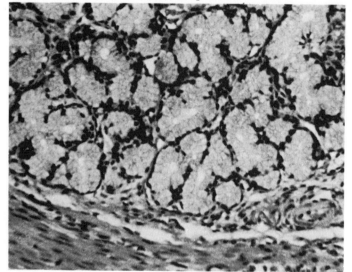

**Fig. 11.11.(b)   Duodenum wall (rat), medium power showing
Brunner's gland in submucosa T.S. ×210**

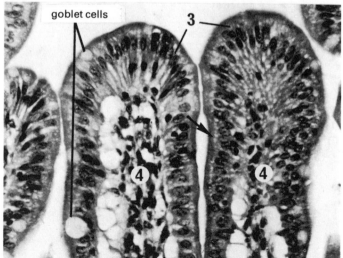

**Fig. 11.11.(c)   Villi of duodenum (rabbit), high power showing
details of columnar surface epithelium (3), with its
striated border (unlabelled arrow), and the lamina
propria (4). ×280**

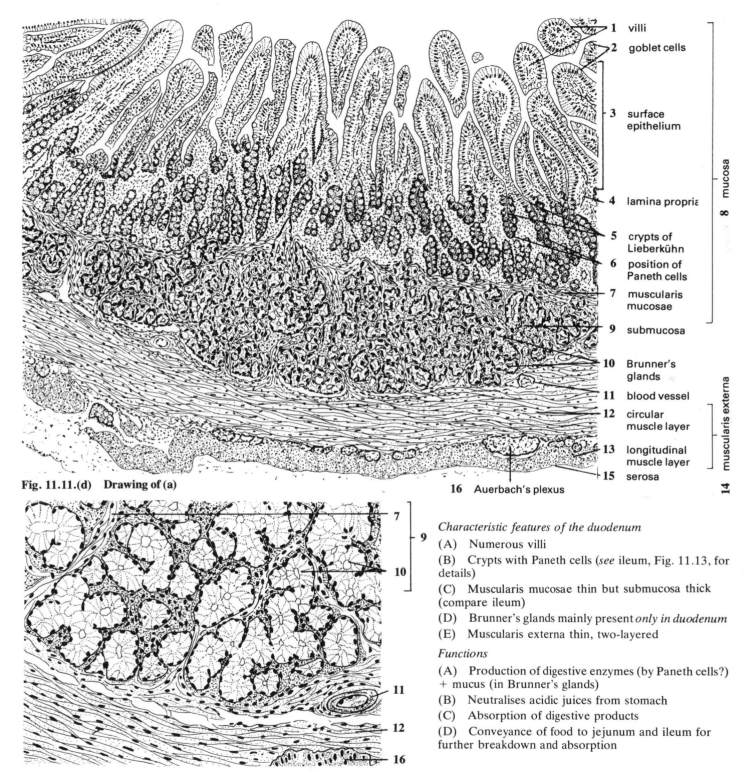

1 villi
2 goblet cells
3 surface epithelium
4 lamina propria
5 crypts of Lieberkühn
6 position of Paneth cells
7 muscularis mucosae
9 submucosa
10 Brunner's glands
11 blood vessel
12 circular muscle layer
13 longitudinal muscle layer
15 serosa
16 Auerbach's plexus
8 mucosa
14 muscularis externa

Fig. 11.11.(d) Drawing of (a)

7
9
10
11
12
16

Fig. 11.11.(e) Drawing of (b)

Characteristic features of the duodenum

(A)   Numerous villi

(B)   Crypts with Paneth cells (*see* ileum, Fig. 11.13, for details)

(C)   Muscularis mucosae thin but submucosa thick (compare ileum)

(D)   Brunner's glands mainly present *only in duodenum*

(E)   Muscularis externa thin, two-layered

Functions

(A)   Production of digestive enzymes (by Paneth cells?) + mucus (in Brunner's glands)

(B)   Neutralises acidic juices from stomach

(C)   Absorption of digestive products

(D)   Conveyance of food to jejunum and ileum for further breakdown and absorption

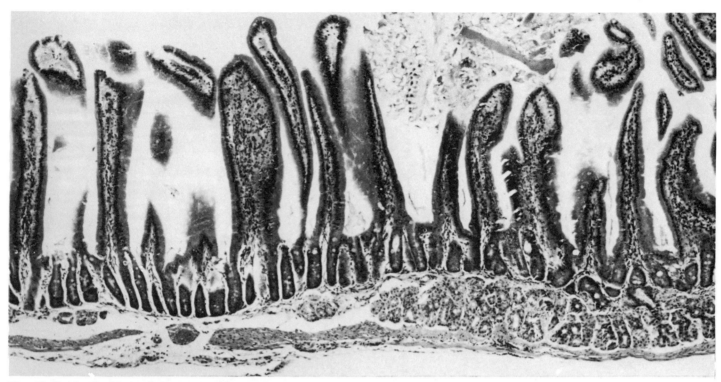

Fig. 11.12.(a) Duodenum/jejunum junction (rat), medium power, L.S. ×110

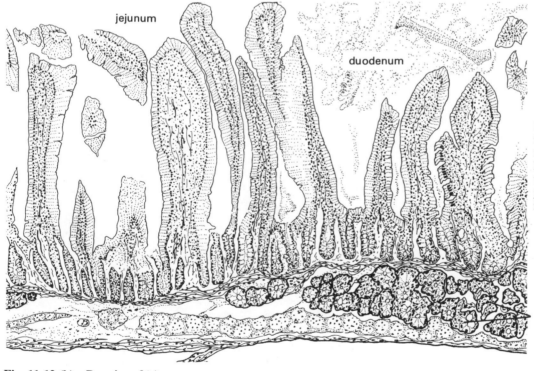

jejunum

duodenum

Labelling as for duodenum and ileum (Figs 11.11 and 11.13) but note gradual disappearance of Brunner's glands (BG) during transition from duodenum to jejunum (= second part of small intestine)

BG

Fig. 11.12.(b) Drawing of (a)

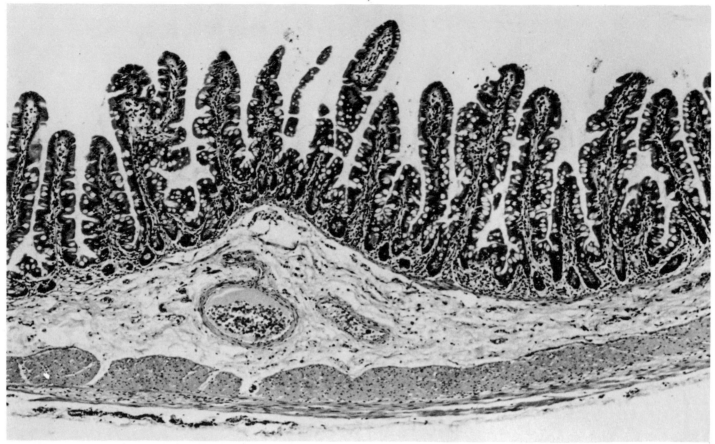

Fig. 11.13.(a)   Ileum (human), low power L.S. ×80

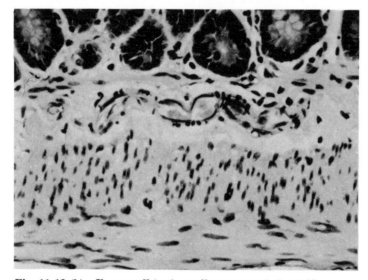

Fig. 11.13.(b)   Ileum wall (rat), medium power, L.S. ×320

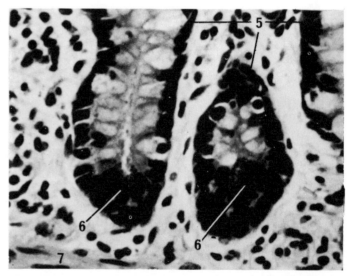

Fig. 11.13.(c)   Paneth cell granules (6) in crypts of Lieberkühn (5) (rat), high power. Phloxine–tartrazine stain. ×560

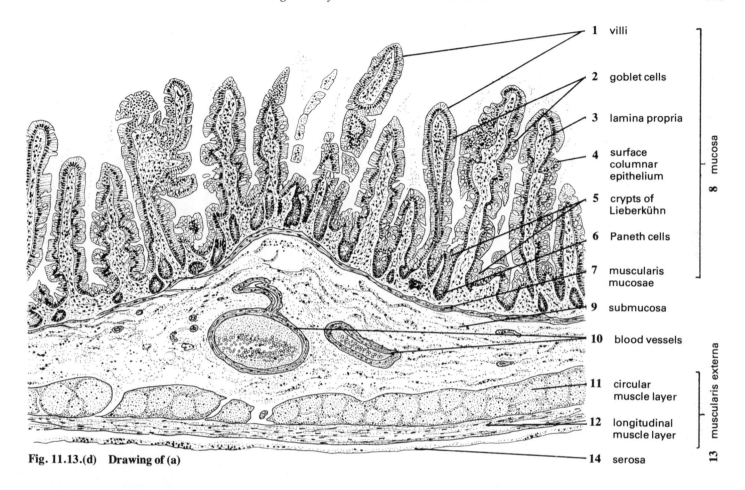

1	villi
2	goblet cells
3	lamina propria
4	surface columnar epithelium
5	crypts of Lieberkühn
6	Paneth cells
7	muscularis mucosae
8	mucosa
9	submucosa
10	blood vessels
11	circular muscle layer
12	longitudinal muscle layer
13	muscularis externa
14	serosa

Fig. 11.13.(d)   Drawing of (a)

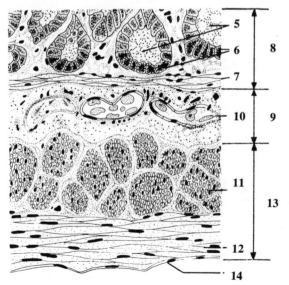

Fig. 11.13.(e)   Drawing of (b)

Characteristic features of ileum

(A)   Numerous villi

(B)   Crypts with Paneth cells (produce enzymes)

(C)   No Brunner's glands in submucosa (compare duodenum)

(D)   Muscularis externa thin, two-layered

(E)   Serosa thin, often difficult to see

Functions

(A)   Production of digestive enzymes and mucus

(B)   Absorption of digestive products

(C)   Conveyance of food to colon

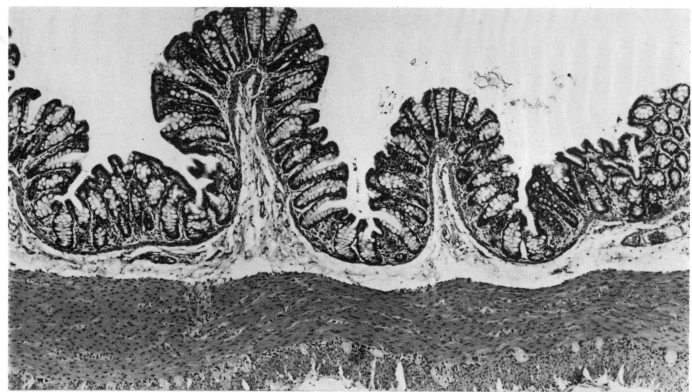

Fig. 11.14.(a)   Large intestine (colon, rat), low power, T.S. ×80

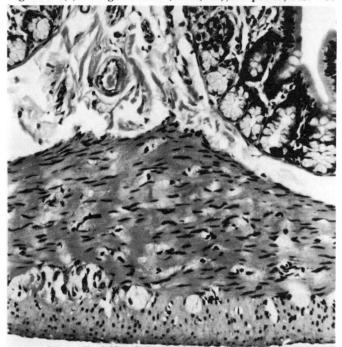

Fig. 11.14.(b)   Large intestine wall (colon, rat), medium power, T.S. ×220

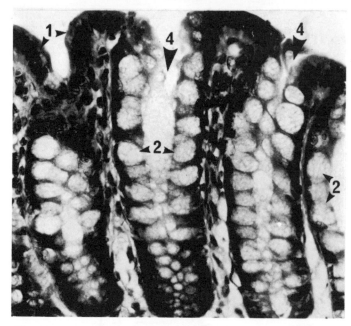

Fig. 11.14.(c)   Crypts of Lieberkühn (4) (colon, rat), high power. Note columnar cells of surface epithelium (1) and numerous goblet cells (2). ×430

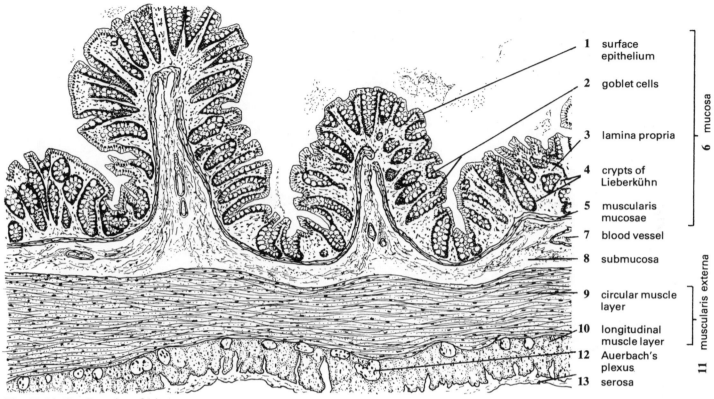

1	surface epithelium
2	goblet cells
3	lamina propria
4	crypts of Lieberkühn
5	muscularis mucosae
7	blood vessel
8	submucosa
9	circular muscle layer
10	longitudinal muscle layer
12	Auerbach's plexus
13	serosa

6 mucosa

11 muscularis externa

Fig. 11.14.(d) Drawing of (a)

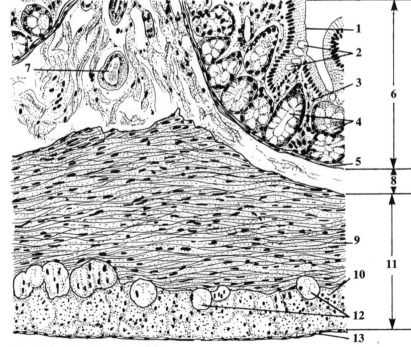

Fig. 11.14.(e) Drawing of (b)

Characteristic features of large intestine

(A) Tube-like crypts (= indentations) but no villi (= finger-like extensions) present — therefore surface smoother than duodenum (Fig. 11.11) and ileum (Fig. 11.13)

(B) Numerous goblet cells in walls of crypts — these clearly distinguish large intestine from pyloric stomach (Fig. 11.9)

(C) Neither Paneth cells nor other specialised cell types present in crypts — therefore resembles pyloric stomach but differs greatly from fundic stomach and ileum

Functions

(A) Absorbs water and salts and conserves body fluids

(B) Moves food remnants to rectum

(C) Stores faeces until expulsion

(D) Some vitamins synthesised by bacteria in lumen

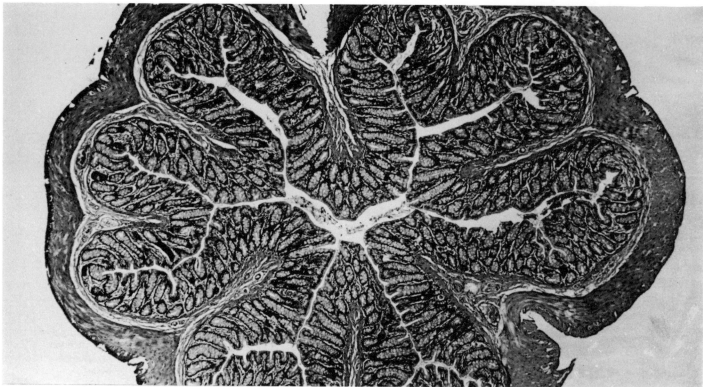

Fig. 11.15.(a)   Rectum (rat), low power, T.S. ×50

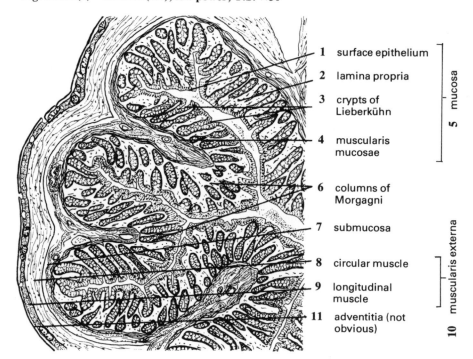

Fig. 11.15.(b)   Drawing of left-hand side of (a)

1   surface epithelium

2   lamina propria

3   crypts of
    Lieberkühn

4   muscularis
    mucosae

5   mucosa

6   columns of
    Morgagni

7   submucosa

8   circular muscle

9   longitudinal
    muscle

11 adventitia (not
    obvious)

10 muscularis externa

Characteristic features of rectum

Structure is very similar to colon (Fig. 11.14) except that large rectal folds are present (columns of Morgagni) and cross-sectional area is much smaller

Functions

(A)   Absorbs water and salts

(B)   Stores and expels faeces

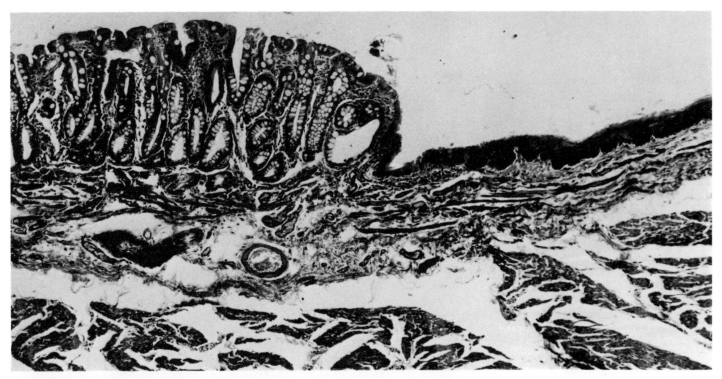

Fig. 11.16.(a)   Anorectal junction (cat), low power, L.S. Masson's triple stain. ×90

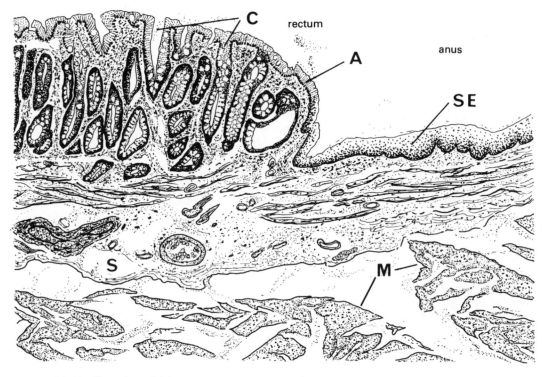

C

rectum

anus

A

SE

S

M

This section clearly shows the transition from the rectum with its crypts of Lieberkühn (C) to the anal canal lined by a stratified squamous epithelium (SE). Note the vascularised submucosa (S), the anal valve (A) and the sphincter muscles (M) of the anus

Fig. 11.16.(b)   Drawing of (a)

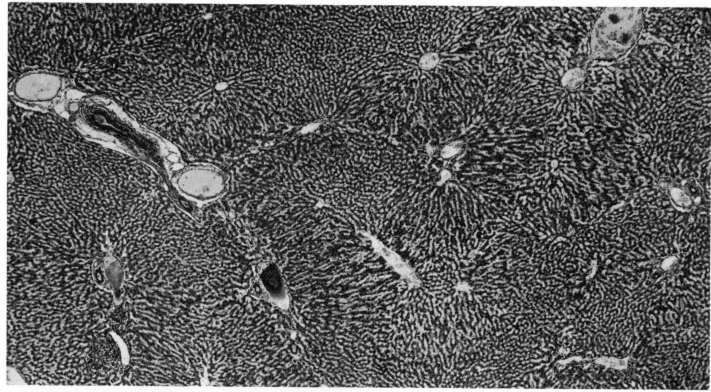

Fig. 11.17.(a)   Liver section (rat), low power. Lobules poorly defined. ×50

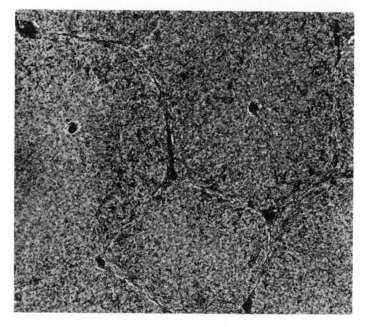

Fig. 11.17.(b)   Liver section (pig), low power showing clearly defined lobules enclosed by connective tissue (= Glisson's capsule). ×50

Characteristic features of the liver

(A)   Lobulate — but only obvious in species (e.g. pig) in which lobules enclosed by a connective tissue sheath (= Glisson's capsule) (*see* (b))

(B)   Hepatic cells radiate out from central vein—like spokes in a wheel

(C)   Tissue of very uniform appearance and not subdivided into layers, in contrast to most organs, e.g. gut, kidney, etc.

(D)   Small groups of vessels (= portal areas) occur at fairly regular intervals between the lobules

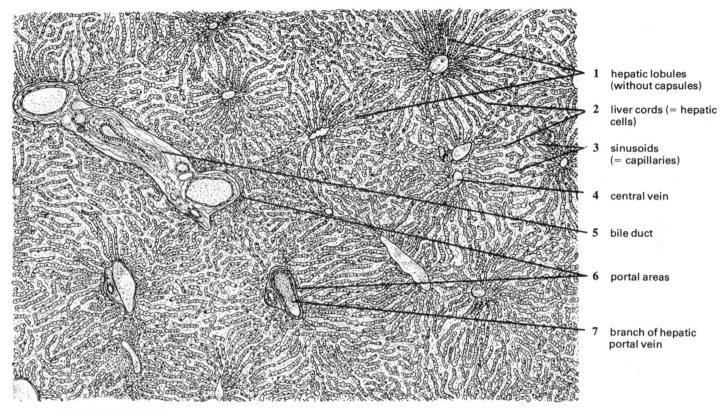

1 hepatic lobules (without capsules)

2 liver cords (= hepatic cells)

3 sinusoids (= capillaries)

4 central vein

5 bile duct

6 portal areas

7 branch of hepatic portal vein

Fig. 11.17.(c) Drawing of (a)

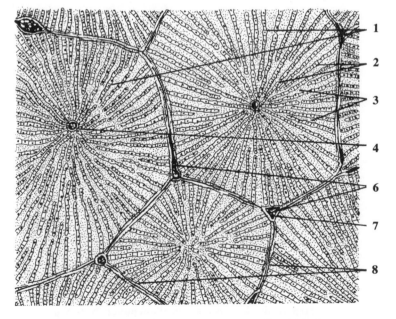

1
2
3
4
6
7
8

Functions

(A) Stores and breaks down carbohydrates and fats
(B) Stores iron and vitamins A, D and B
(C) Forms urea from excess protein
(D) Synthesises bile and plasma proteins
(E) Detoxifies harmful substances, e.g. drugs
(F) Produces heat

Fig. 11.17.(d) Drawing of (b) showing clearly defined lobules enclosed by connective tissue (8) (= Glisson's capsule)

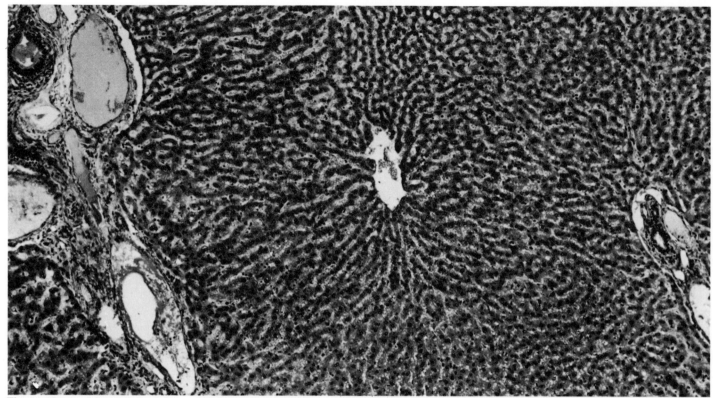

Fig. 11.18.(a)   Liver section (rat), medium power, showing details of one lobule. ×130. *N.B.* No connective tissue capsule around
           lobule

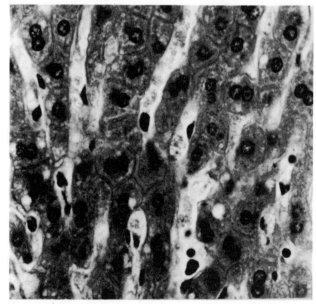

Fig. 11.18.(b)   Liver section (rat), high power, showing
           details of hepatic cells, bile canaliculi and
           position of fixed phagocytes (= Kupffer
           cells). ×430

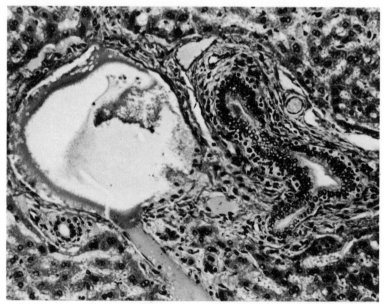

Fig. 11.18.(c)   Hepatic portal area (rat), medium power. Note hepatic
           portal vein and bile ducts. ×240. *N.B.* Hepatic artery
           not obvious here

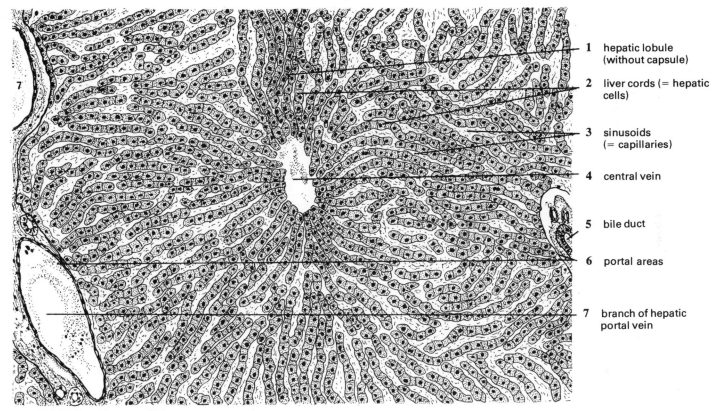

Fig. 11.18.(d)   **Drawing of (a)**

1 hepatic lobule
   (without capsule)

2 liver cords (= hepatic
   cells)

3 sinusoids
   (= capillaries)

4 central vein

5 bile duct

6 portal areas

7 branch of hepatic
   portal vein

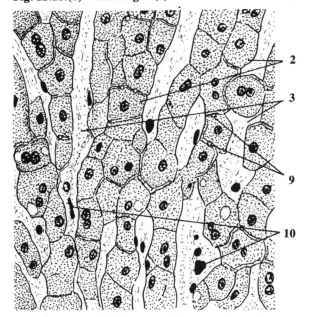

Fig. 11.18.(e)   **Drawing of (b) showing details of hepatic
cells (2), bile canaliculi (9) and position of
fixed phagocytes (10) (= Kupffer cells)**

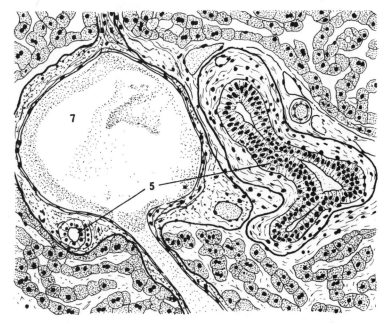

Fig. 11.18.(f)   **Drawing of (c) showing hepatic portal vein (7) and bile
ducts (5)**

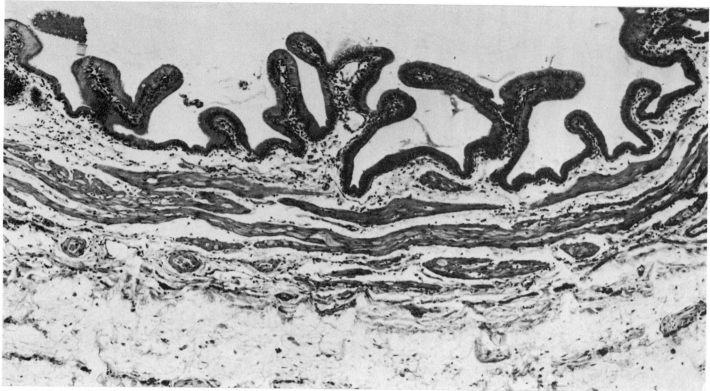

Fig. 11.19.(a)   Gall bladder (human), low power, section. ×90

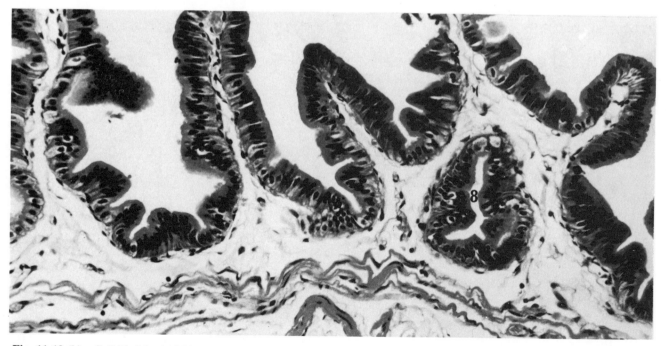

**Fig. 11.19.(b)   Gall bladder (rabbit), medium power, showing columnar cells of lining folds. Note fold cut in section (8)
resembling gland, and serosa. Section. ×250**

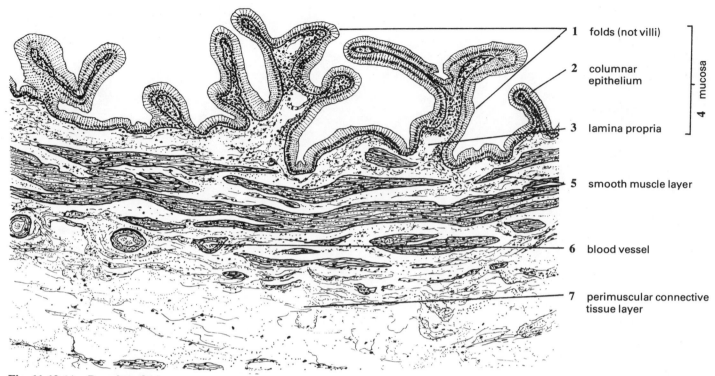

1 folds (not villi)

2 columnar epithelium

4 mucosa

3 lamina propria

5 smooth muscle layer

6 blood vessel

7 perimuscular connective tissue layer

Fig. 11.19.(c)   Drawing of (a)

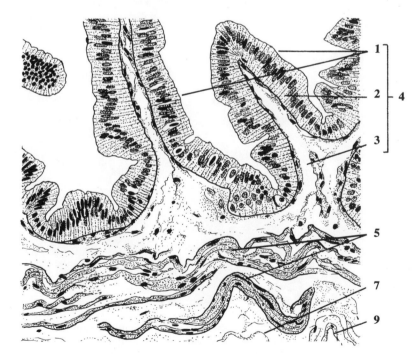

Fig. 11.19.(d)   Drawing of (b) showing columnar cells (2) of lining folds (1). Note serosa (9)

Characteristic features of gall bladder

(A)   Superficially resembles gut, but epithelium = one cell type with no goblet cells or gland cells present

(B)   Muscularis mucosae, submucosa and muscularis externa absent

(C)   Smooth muscle layer composed of loose network of fibres, in contrast to compact muscularis externa of gut

Functions

(A)   Stores, concentrates and expels bile into duodenum via bile duct

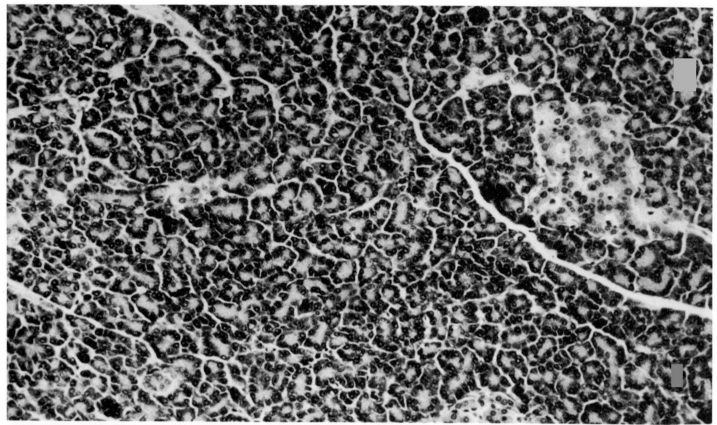

Fig. 11.20.(a)   Pancreas (rat), low power, section. ×150

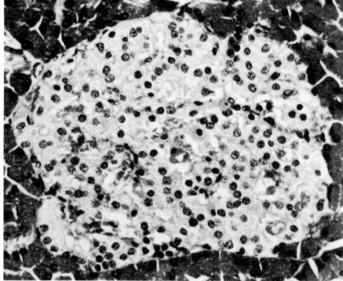

**Fig. 11.20.(b)   Pancreas (rat), medium power of islet of
Langerhans stained with haematoxylin and eosin,
which fails to differentiate between various cell
types in islet. ×300**

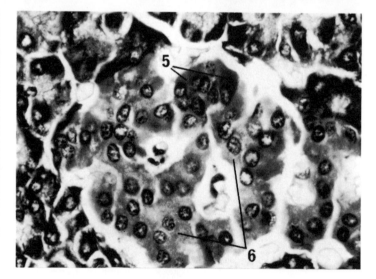

**Fig. 11.20.(c)   Islet of Langerhans (rat), high power showing
alpha cells (5) staining darker than the more
common, central, beta cells (6) after using
Gomori haematoxylin–phloxine technique. × 650**

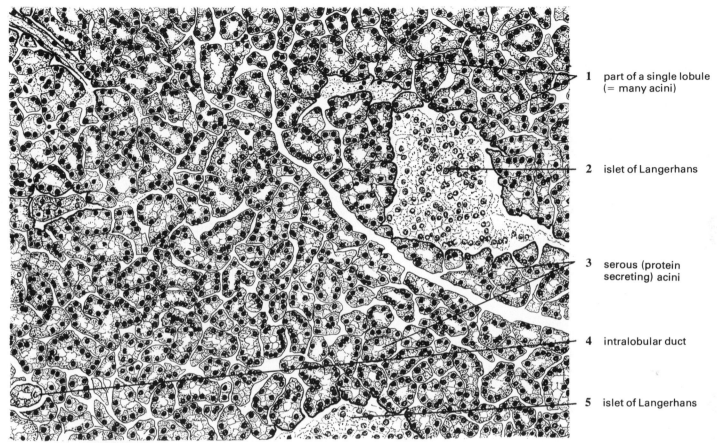

1 part of a single lobule (= many acini)

2 islet of Langerhans

3 serous (protein secreting) acini

4 intralobular duct

5 islet of Langerhans

Fig. 11.20.(d)   Drawing of (a)

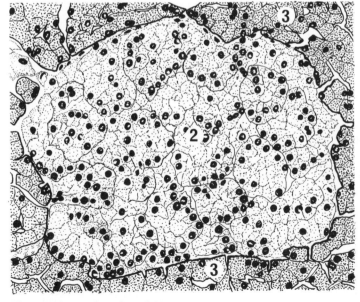

Fig. 11.20.(e)   Drawing of (b)

Characteristic features of pancreas

(A)   Homogeneous gland of numerous serous (= protein secreting) acini (= groups of gland cells)

(B)   Round, lighter-staining areas (= islets) scattered throughout section

(C)   Structure similar to serous salivary glands (e.g. parotid, *see* Fig. 11.4) except islets present and ducts less distinct

Functions

(A)   Acini (= exocrine part) secrete alkaline juice into duodenum to neutralise acid of stomach, and contains trypsin, chymotrypsin, carboxypeptidase (digest protein), amylases (digest carbohydrate), lipases (digest fat) and nucleases (digest nucleic acids)

(B)   Islets of Langerhans (= endocrine part) secrete hormones, insulin (↓ blood glucose, produced by beta cells) and glucagon (↑ blood glucose, produced by alpha cells)

12 Urinary System*

The urinary system consists of a *pair of kidneys,* the *ureters,* the *bladder* and the *urethra.* The kidneys filter the blood and produce urine. The ureters transport the urine to the bladder where it is stored and from which it eventually passes to the outside via the urethra. In the male, semen is also discharged through the urethra. Micrographs of the kidneys are given in Figs 12.2 to 12.4, and of the ureter and bladder in Figs 12.5 and 12.6 respectively.

12.1 KIDNEYS

The kidney (Figs 12.1–12.4) is bean-shaped with an indentation, the *hilus,* on one side, from which the ureter arises. When the cut surface of a whole kidney is viewed with the naked eye, an outer dark-red layer, the *cortex,* can be distinguished from an inner lighter region, the

medulla. Kidney structure, however, is not always that simple, and in different species may be complicated by the arrangement of the medulla into many *pyramids* and also by the expansion of the upper end of the ureter to form the *pelvis,* which may branch to form the *major calyces* which in turn may give rise to many *minor calyces (see* Fig. 12.1). Gross examination of histological sections of the kidney with the naked eye may well alleviate some of the problems of interpretation and allow the student to determine the plane of sectioning. The section should ideally pass through the cortex, medulla and pelvis of the kidney. The complexity of the structure of kidney thus varies greatly from one species to another. The simplest and most easily interpreted structure is that of the *unilobular kidney,* found in rats, rabbits, guinea pigs, etc., while the *multilobular kidney* of man is much more complex.

In the unilobular kidney *(see* Fig. 12.1), the whole

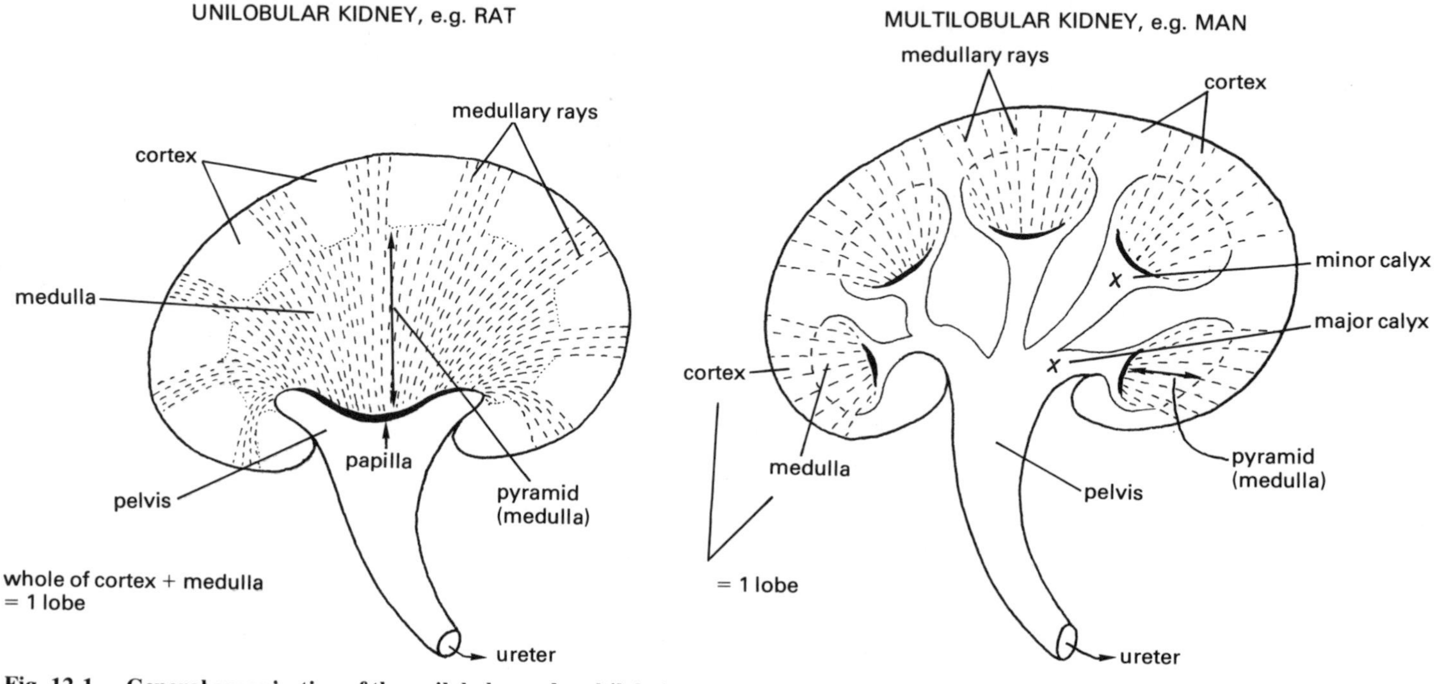

UNILOBULAR KIDNEY, e.g. RAT

MULTILOBULAR KIDNEY, e.g. MAN

Fig. 12.1. **General organisation of the unilobular and multilobular types of kidney**

*See Fig. 3.1 for location of parts.

kidney contains just one lobe. A lobe is formed by the medulla, which is pyramid-shaped and hence called the *pyramid,* together with the cortex, which covers the base of the pyramid. The point of the pyramid, or the *papilla,* empties into a single pelvis. In the multilobular kidney of man, many lobes, and hence pyramids and papillae, are found, and since all the papillae cannot possibly empty directly into the pelvis, this subdivides. The larger branches are the *major calyces,* and these branch further to form the *minor calyces,* each of which caps a papilla of a pyramid.

The functional unit of the kidney is the *nephron* or *excretory tubule* (*see* Fig. 12.2). This consists of a *knot of blood vessels* (= afferent and efferent arterioles), the *glomerulus,* which rests in the thin expanded end of the nephron, called the *Bowman's capsule,* from which a long tube composed of the *proximal convoluted tubule,* the *loop of Henle* and the *distal convoluted tubule* passes before emptying into the *collecting tubule* which discharges into the pelvis of the ureter. The glomerulus plus the Bowman's capsule form the filtration unit of the kidney, and together are termed the *renal* or *Malpighian corpuscle.* The filtrate passes under pressure from the glomerulus into the Bowman's capsule and thence into the main body of the tubule. During its passage towards the collecting duct, substances of use to the body, such as salts, glucose, water, etc., are *selectively reabsorbed* back into the blood by the wall of the tubule. Renal corpuscles are confined to the cortex, which also contains light-coloured extensions of medullary tissue originating from the base of the pyramids and called *medullary rays.* These rays contain branches of the collecting tubules and the loops of Henle, which make up the main substance of the medulla.

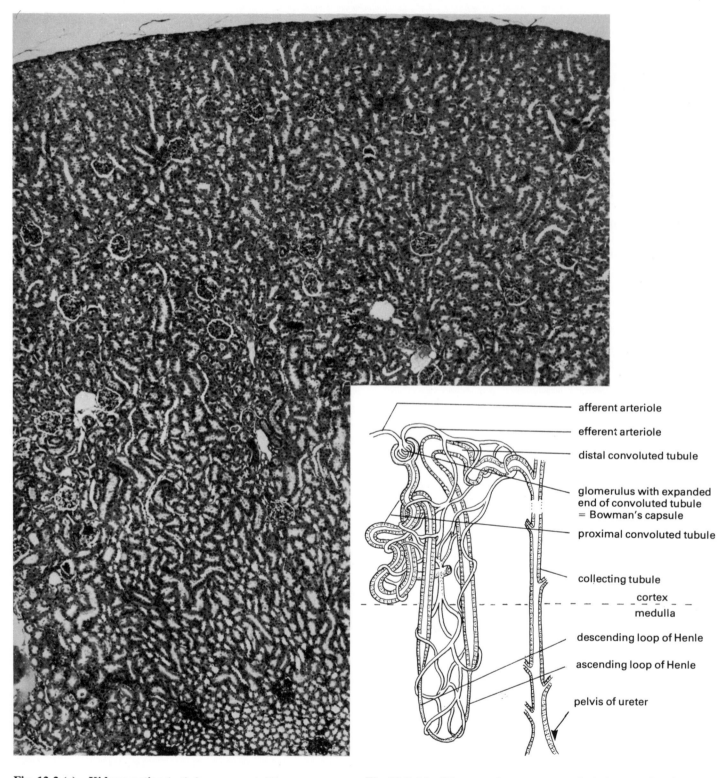

Fig. 12.2.(a)   Kidney section (rat), low power. ×45

Fig. 12.2.(b)   Diagram of an excretory tubule (= a nephron)

afferent arteriole

efferent arteriole

distal convoluted tubule

glomerulus with expanded
end of convoluted tubule
= Bowman's capsule

proximal convoluted tubule

collecting tubule

cortex

medulla

descending loop of Henle

ascending loop of Henle

pelvis of ureter

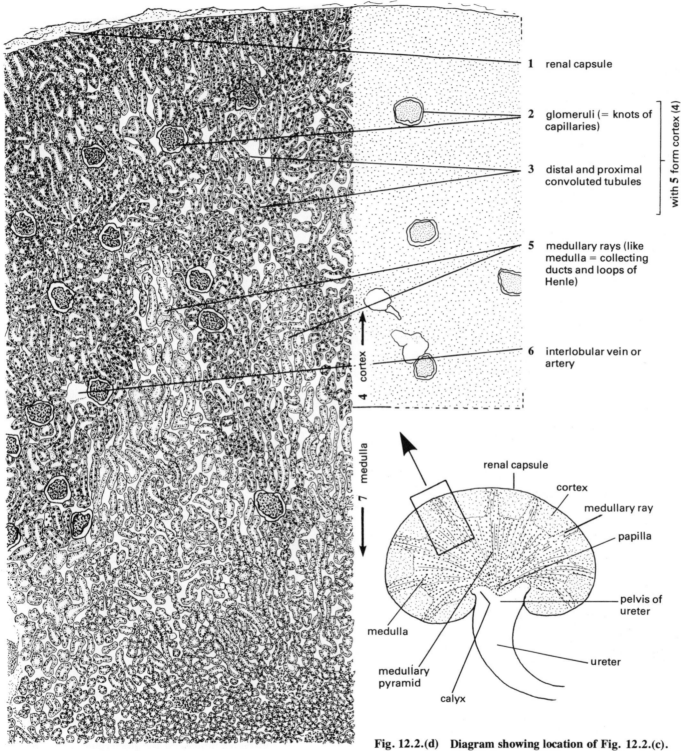

1 renal capsule

2 glomeruli (= knots of capillaries)

3 distal and proximal convoluted tubules

with 5 form cortex (4)

5 medullary rays (like medulla = collecting ducts and loops of Henle)

6 interlobular vein or artery

cortex

4

7 medulla

Fig. 12.2.(c)   Drawing of (a)

renal capsule

cortex

medullary ray

papilla

pelvis of ureter

ureter

medulla

medullary pyramid

calyx

**Fig. 12.2.(d)   Diagram showing location of Fig. 12.2.(c).
N.B. Only one medullary pyramid and one lobe
present in rat, guinea pig, etc.**

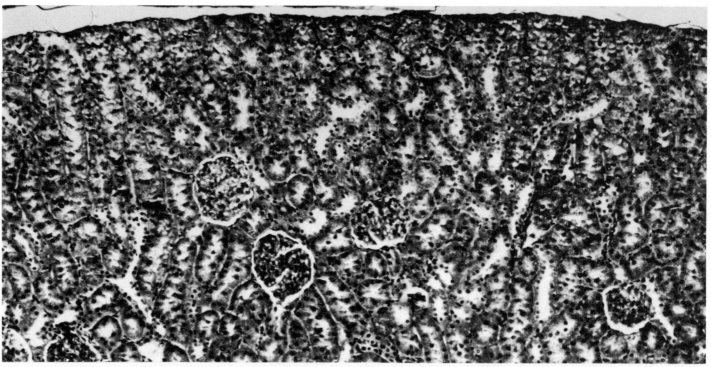

Fig. 12.3.(a)   Kidney section (rat), medium power of outer cortex. ×160

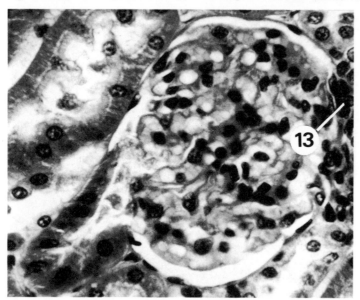

Fig. 12.3.(b)   Kidney (rat), high power of glomerulus which is surrounded by the Bowman's capsule. Note brush border of proximal convoluted tubules, thinner-walled distal convoluted tubules, and macula densa (13) (= thickening of wall of distal convoluted tubule in region of contact with afferent arteriole of glomerulus). ×650

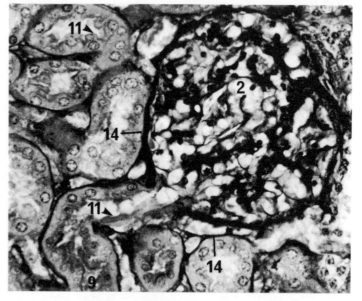

Fig. 12.3.(c)   Kidney (guinea pig), high power stained by periodic acid Schiff technique to show deeply staining polysaccharides in basement membranes (14). Note brush border (11) of proximal convoluted tubules (9) and glomerulus (2). ×350

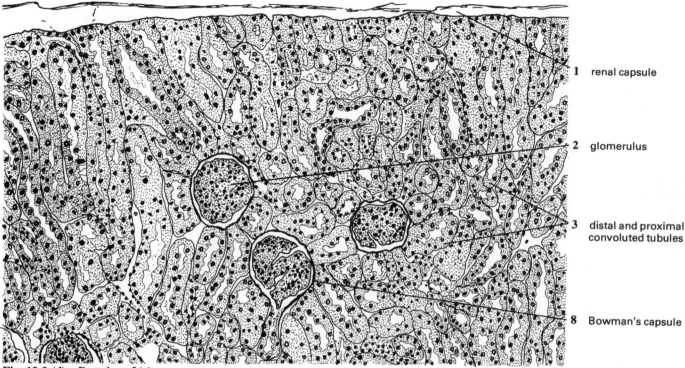

1 renal capsule

2 glomerulus

3 distal and proximal convoluted tubules

8 Bowman's capsule

Fig. 12.3.(d) Drawing of (a)

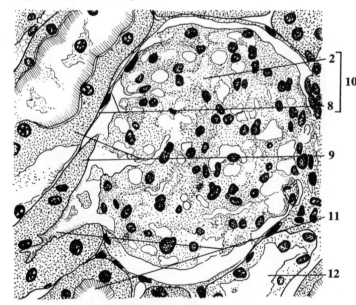

Fig. 12.3.(e) Drawing of (b) showing glomerulus (2) surrounded by the Bowman's capsule (8) (= blind end of convoluted tubule (9) and with glomerulus forms renal or Malpighian corpuscle (10)). Note brush border (11) of proximal convoluted tubules (9) and thinner-walled distal convoluted tubules (12)

Characteristic features of kidney

(A)   Bean-shaped and composed of numerous tubules

(B)   Divided into outer cortex (= granular) and inner medulla (= striated)

(C)   Cortex contains numerous knots of blood vessels (= glomeruli)

(D)   Medulla composed of one, e.g. rat, rabbit, or many, e.g. man, pyramids or lobes (lobe = medullary pyramid + overlying cap of cortical tissue)

Functions

(A)   Excretion—filters blood and produces urine which contains nitrogenous waste, excess salts, etc.

(B)   Maintains homeostasis of body by selective reabsorption of ions, glucose and water from urine across tubule walls

(C)   Produces renin which is involved in regulating blood pressure and raising erythrocyte numbers

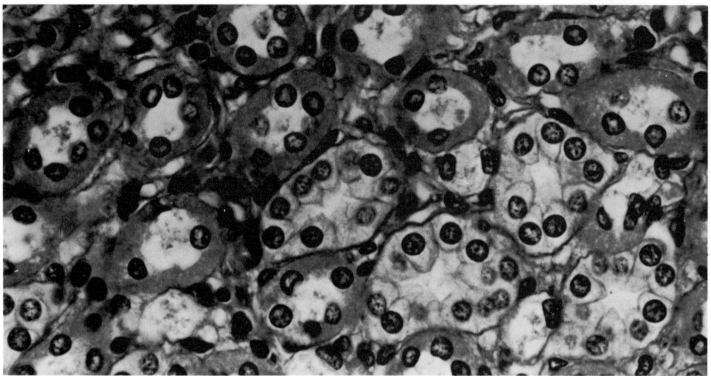

Fig. 12.4.(a)   Kidney section (rabbit), high power of medulla. ×900

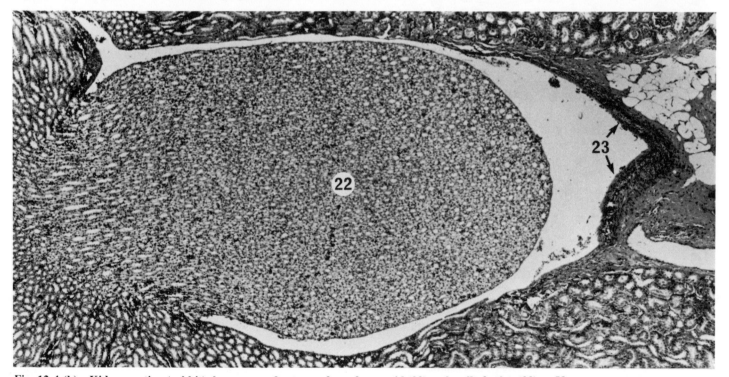

Fig. 12.4.(b)   Kidney section (rabbit), low power of outer surface of pyramid (22) and wall of calyx (23). ×58

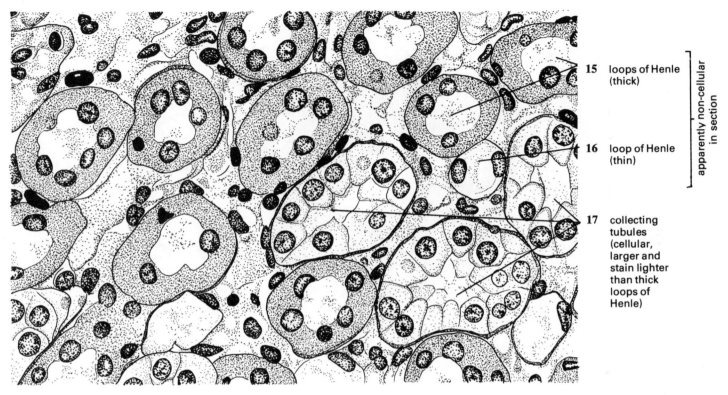

15 loops of Henle (thick)

16 loop of Henle (thin)

apparently non-cellular in section

17 collecting tubules (cellular, larger and stain lighter than thick loops of Henle)

Fig. 12.4.(c)   Drawing of (a)

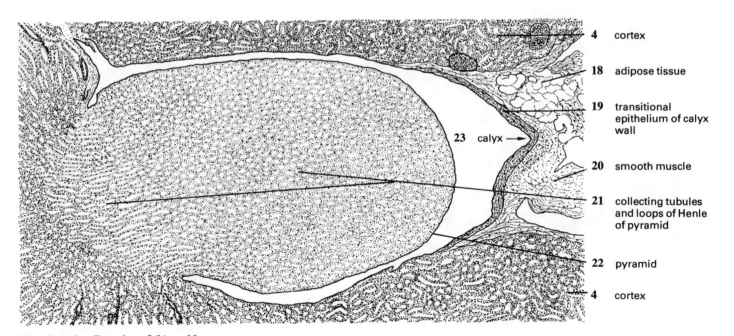

4 cortex

18 adipose tissue

19 transitional epithelium of calyx wall

23 calyx →

20 smooth muscle

21 collecting tubules and loops of Henle of pyramid

22 pyramid

4 cortex

Fig. 12.4.(d)   Drawing of (b). ×46

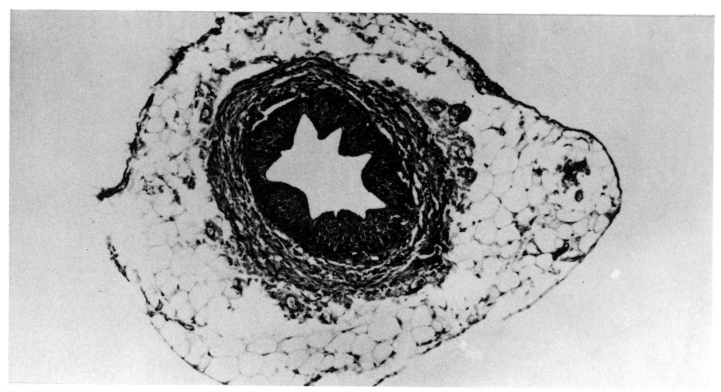

Fig. 12.5.(a)   Ureter (cat), low power T.S. Surrounded by adipose tissue (fat). ×100

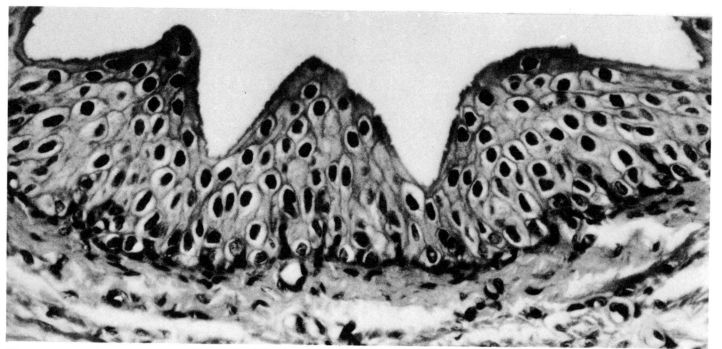

Fig. 12.5.(b)   Transitional epithelium of ureter (cat), high power. Note underlying layer of smooth muscle interspersed by connective tissue. × 650

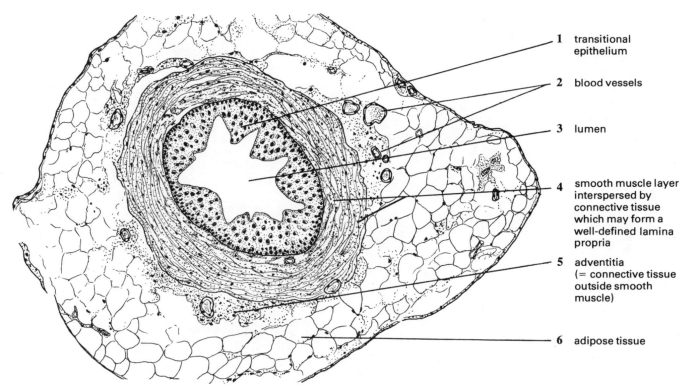

1 transitional epithelium

2 blood vessels

3 lumen

4 smooth muscle layer interspersed by connective tissue which may form a well-defined lamina propria

5 adventitia (= connective tissue outside smooth muscle)

6 adipose tissue

Fig. 12.5.(c)   Drawing of (a)

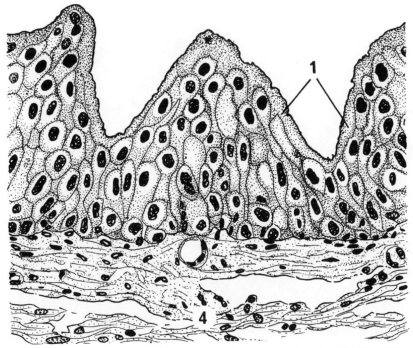

Fig. 12.5.(d)   Drawing of middle region of (b). Transitional epithelium (1), smooth muscle layer (4)

Characteristic features of ureter

(A)   Star-shaped lumen

(B)   Transitional epithelium (therefore not gut)

(C)   Thick smooth muscle layer (with longitudinal and circular fibres)

(D)   Surrounded by adipose tissue

Functions

(A)   Propels and conveys urine to bladder

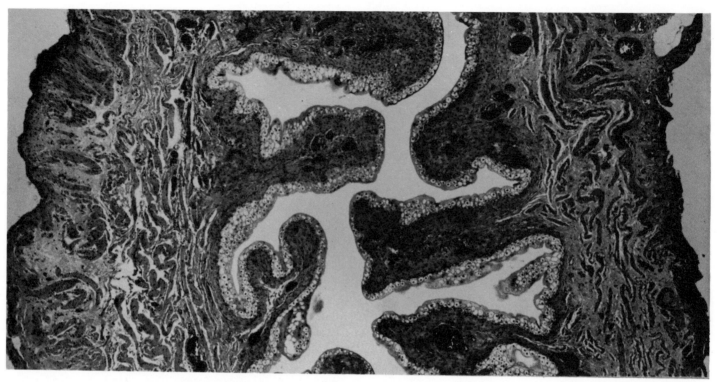

Fig. 12.6.(a)   Urinary bladder (rabbit), low-power section. ×60

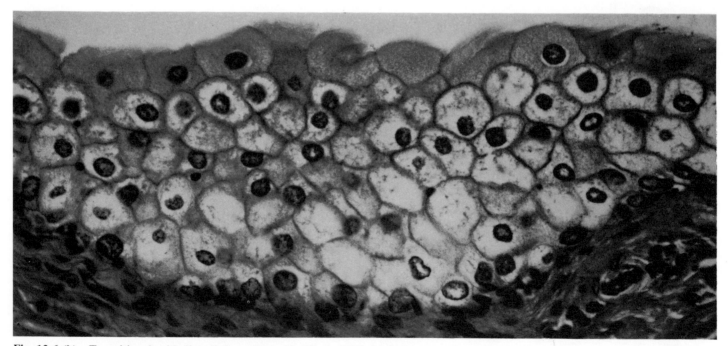

Fig. 12.6.(b)   Transitional epithelium lining urinary bladder (rabbit), high-power section. Note rounded cells of contracted bladder (= empty) and connective tissue. ×600

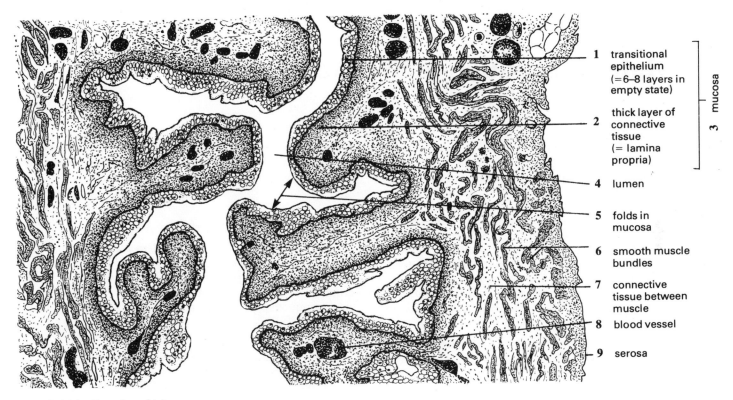

1 transitional epithelium (=6–8 layers in empty state)

2 thick layer of connective tissue (= lamina propria)

3 mucosa

4 lumen

5 folds in mucosa

6 smooth muscle bundles

7 connective tissue between muscle

8 blood vessel

9 serosa

Fig. 12.6.(c) Drawing of (a)

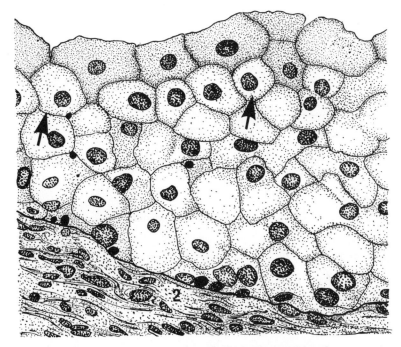

Fig. 12.6.(d) Drawing of (b). Note rounded cells (arrows) of contracted bladder (= empty) and connective tissue (2)

Characteristic features of urinary bladder

Superficially resembles gut, but in contrast:

(A) Transitional epithelium lines lumen

(B) Smooth muscle coat does not appear to be composed of definite layers but of small, randomly arranged bundles

(C) Much connective tissue separates bundles of muscle

Functions

Collects and stores urine excreted from kidneys via ureters and discharges it into urethra → outside

13 Male Reproductive System

The male reproductive system functions to *produce* and *transfer spermatozoa* to the female for fertilisation of the mature egg cell. It also synthesises the male sex hormone, *testosterone,* which influences the development of the secondary sex characteristics and organs at puberty, e.g. facial hair, deepening of voice, enlargement of penis, etc.

The male reproductive system (Fig. 13.1) consists of a pair of *testes* for sperm and testosterone production, a *number of ducts,* e.g. the *epididymis* and *ductus deferens* for transport of the semen to the penis, *accessory glands,* i.e. two *seminal vesicles,* one (man) or two (rat) *prostate gland(s)* and two *bulbourethral glands* which add their

secretion to the spermatozoa to produce the fluid semen, and a copulatory organ or *penis* which introduces the semen to the female reproductive system.

13.1   TESTES

Each testis (Fig. 13.2) is enclosed in a connective tissue capsule, the *tunica albuginea,* and is subdivided by thin fibrous septa into approximately *250 lobules.* Each lobule contains 1–4 highly folded *seminiferous tubules* which lie in a connective tissue matrix also containing blood and

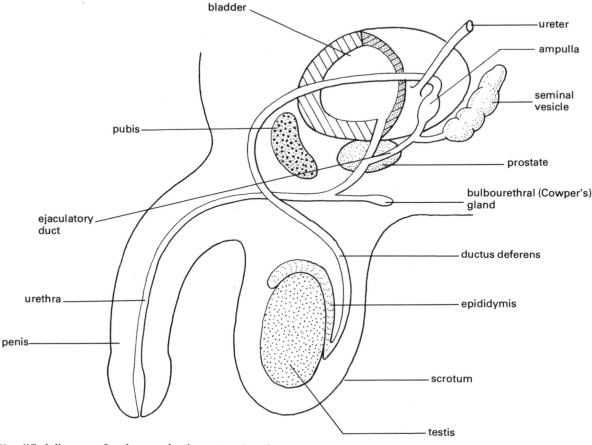

Fig. 13.1.   Simplified diagram of male reproductive system (man)

150

lymph vessels, nerves and the testosterone-synthesising *interstitial cells of Leydig* (endocrine portion of testis).

The seminiferous tubules are lined by *stratified epithelium* composed of two types of cells. One cell type, the *Sertoli cell,* is supportive, while the other, the *spermatogenic cell,* produces the *spermatozoa.* Sertoli cells are often difficult to identify in histological sections but characteristically are tall cells attached to the basement membrane, are broad at the base and taper towards the lumen of the tubule, have mature spermatozoa embedded in their apices and have a lighter-staining, larger nucleus than the surrounding spermatogenic cells. They occur scattered between large numbers of spermatogenic cells and probably function to support and nourish the developing spermatozoa, and may also have an endocrine function. The spermatogenic cells occur in various stages of differentiation from *spermatogonia,* adjacent to the basement membrane and in various stages of *meiosis* and *mitosis,* → primary and secondary *spermatocytes* → *spermatids* → *spermatozoa* free in the lumen. Different sections of the seminiferous tubules are in various stages of *spermatogenesis* and not all regions contain mature spermatozoa in their lumens.

13.2 DUCTS

The seminiferous tubules empty via the efferent ductules into a highly coiled tube, the *ductus epididymis* (Fig. 13.3), which partially covers the testis and serves to *store the sperm.* The epididymis is lined by a *pseudostratified columnar epithelium* which has stereocilia on its free surface. Sperm is ejected from the epididymis to the *ductus deferens* (Fig. 13.4) which conveys it by contractions of its muscular coat to the *ampulla* of the *ductus deferens* and the duct of the *seminal vesicle* which together are termed the *ejaculatory duct.* The two ejaculatory ducts empty into the *urethra* which conveys the sperm into and along the *penis* (Fig. 13.1).

13.3 ACCESSORY GLANDS

In man, these are the *seminal vesicles* (Fig. 13.5), *prostate gland* (Fig. 13.6) and *bulbourethral glands.* They are associated with the various ducts (described above) and add their secretion to the semen during ejaculation. These secretions either provide an energy source for the sperm (= fructose from seminal vesicles), dilute the semen and stimulate sperm movement (= prostate gland) or lubricate the urethra (= bulbourethral glands). In the rat, the seminal vesicles are very large and closely associated with two additional glands, the *coagulating glands.*

13.4 PENIS

This consists of a mass of spongy tissue into which blood is pumped to make it erect for conveyance of the sperm into the vagina.

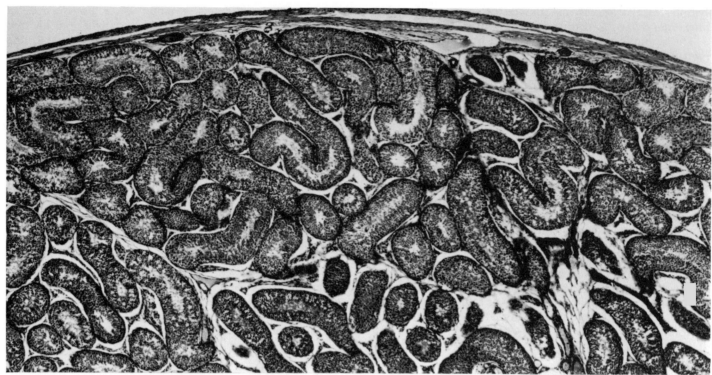

Fig. 13.2.(a)   Testis (rat), low-power section. ×55

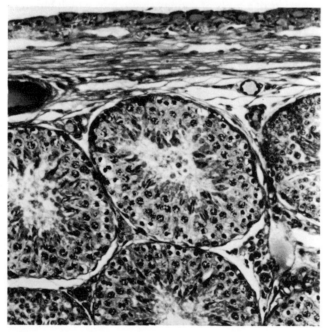

Fig. 13.2.(b)   Testis (rat), medium-power section of several seminiferous tubules. ×230

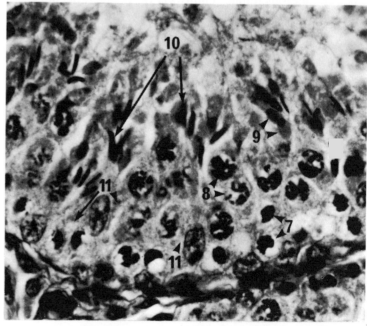

Fig. 13.2.(c)   Wall of seminiferous tubule (rat), high power. Note heads of mature spermatozoa (10) embedded in apices of Sertoli cells (11). Spermatogonia (7), primary spermatocytes (8), spermatids (9). ×830

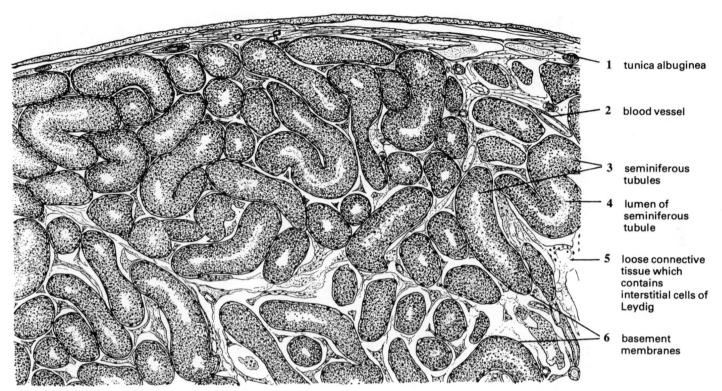

1	tunica albuginea
2	blood vessel
3	seminiferous tubules
4	lumen of seminiferous tubule
5	loose connective tissue which contains interstitial cells of Leydig
6	basement membranes

Fig. 13.2.(d)   Drawing of (a)

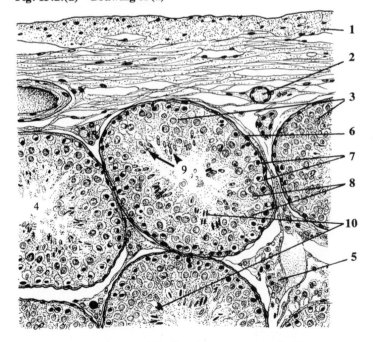

Characteristic features of testis

(A)   Many tubules present in section

(B)   Thick outer capsule (tunica albuginea)

(C)   Many meiotic/mitotic figures visible in walls of tubules

(D)   Spermatozoa present in tubules

Functions

(A)   Production of male gametes (spermatozoa) in tubules

(B)   Production of male sex hormone, testosterone, by interstitial cells

Fig. 13.2.(e)   Drawing of (b) showing spermatogonia (7), primary spermatocytes (8), spermatids (9) and spermatozoa (10) in lumen (4)

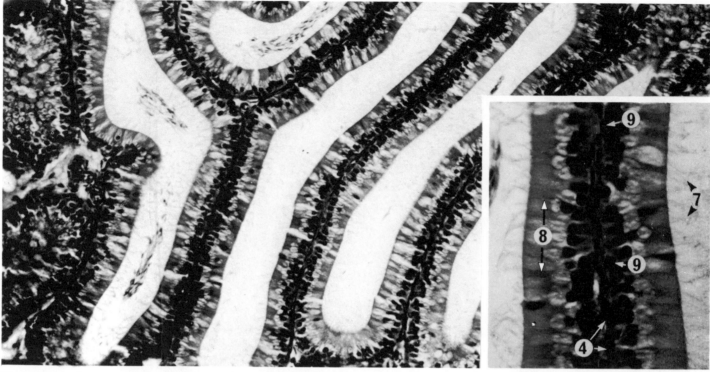

Fig. 13.3.(a)   Ductus epididymis (rat), medium power, section. ×230

Fig. 13.3.(b)   'Ciliated' pseudostratified columnar epithelium of ductus epididymis (rat), high power. Note stereocilia (7), columnar cells (8), basal cells (9) and position of smooth muscle (4). ×500

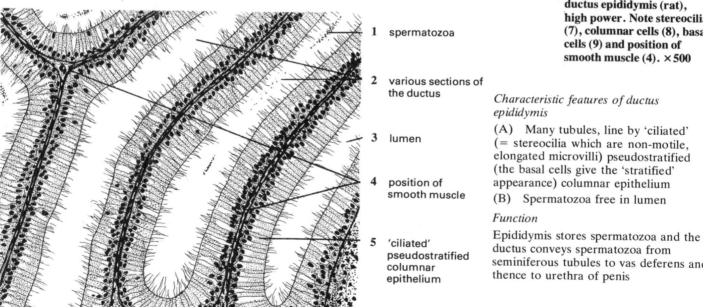

1 spermatozoa

2 various sections of the ductus

3 lumen

4 position of smooth muscle

5 'ciliated' pseudostratified columnar epithelium

6 connective tissue

Fig. 13.3.(c)   Drawing of (a)

Characteristic features of ductus epididymis

(A)   Many tubules, line by 'ciliated' (= stereocilia which are non-motile, elongated microvilli) pseudostratified (the basal cells give the 'stratified' appearance) columnar epithelium

(B)   Spermatozoa free in lumen

Function

Epididymis stores spermatozoa and the ductus conveys spermatozoa from seminiferous tubules to vas deferens and thence to urethra of penis

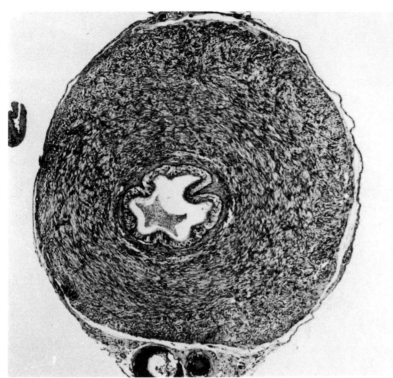

Fig. 13.4.(a)   Ductus deferens (rabbit), low power, T.S. ×50

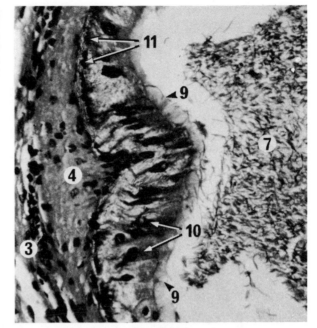

Fig. 13.4.(b)   'Ciliated' pseudostratified columnar epithelium of ductus deferens (rabbit), high power. Note spermatozoa (7), stereocilia (9), columnar cells (10), basal cells (11), connective tissue (4) and inner longitudinal smooth muscle layer (3). ×370

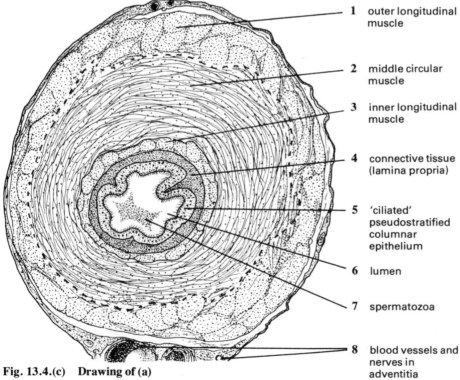

Fig. 13.4.(c)   Drawing of (a)

1 outer longitudinal muscle

2 middle circular muscle

3 inner longitudinal muscle

4 connective tissue (lamina propria)

5 'ciliated' pseudostratified columnar epithelium

6 lumen

7 spermatozoa

8 blood vessels and nerves in adventitia

Characteristic features of ductus deferens

(A)   Tubular and lined by 'ciliated' (= stereocilia as in epididymis) pseudostratified columnar epithelium which distinguishes it from ureter

(B)   Thick, smooth muscle coat

(C)   Narrow lumen containing spermatozoa also distinguishes it from ureter

Function

Muscular wall contracts and propels spermatozoa into urethra of penis

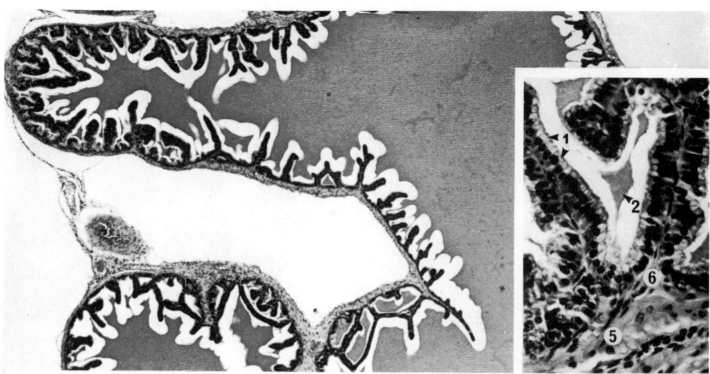

Fig. 13.5.(a)   Seminal vesicle (rat), low power, section. ×60

Fig. 13.5.(b)   **Much-folded pseudostratified columnar epithelium of seminal vesicle (rat), high power. Note secretion (2), columnar cells (1), thin layer of connective tissue (6 = lamina propria) and smooth muscle (5). ×350**

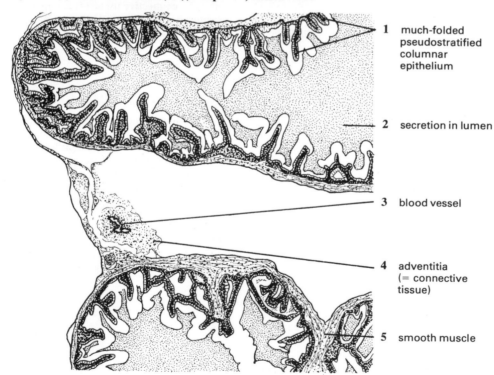

1   much-folded pseudostratified columnar epithelium

2   secretion in lumen

3   blood vessel

4   adventitia (= connective tissue)

5   smooth muscle

Fig. 13.5.(c)   **Drawing of (a)**

Characteristic features of seminal vesicle

(A)   Sac-like structure

(B)   Much-folded pseudostratified columnar epithelium

(C)   Clear secretion in large lumen

Function

Produces a thick secretion which is discharged into the vas deferens and contains fructose which provides the energy source for the spermatozoa

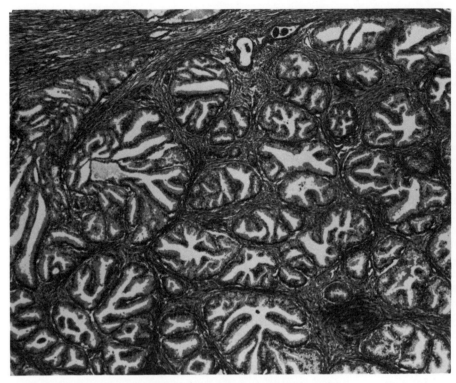

Fig. 13.6.(a)   Prostate gland (human), low power, section. × 60

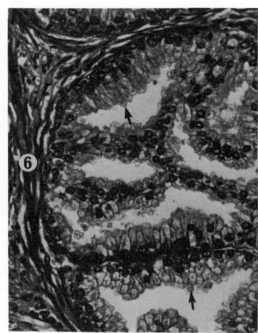

Fig. 13.6.(b)   **Pseudostratified columnar epithelium of alveolar glands in prostate (human), high power. Note columnar cells which bulge into the lumen in places (arrows), and smooth muscle fibres (6). ×350**

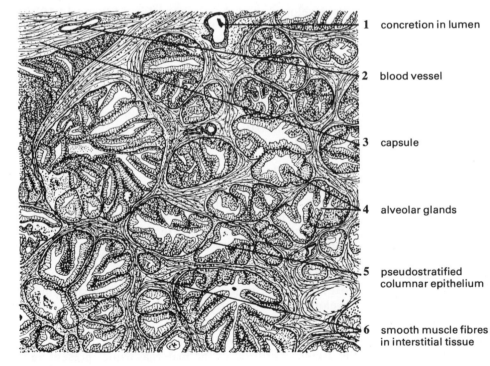

Fig. 13.6.(c)   **Drawing of (a)**

1   concretion in lumen

2   blood vessel

3   capsule

4   alveolar glands

5   pseudostratified columnar epithelium

6   smooth muscle fibres in interstitial tissue

Characteristic features of prostate

(A)   Composed of numerous irregular, tubular glands

(B)   No spermatozoa or stereocilia present

(C)   Dense concretions often present in lumen

(D)   Abundance of muscle fibres present between glands

(E)   Thick capsule

Functions

Produces an acidic secretion which dilutes semen and stimulates movements of spermatozoa

14 Female Reproductive System*

The female reproductive system consists of a pair of *ovaries,* which produce the egg cells (ova) and various hormones, a pair of *fallopian tubes* (= oviducts or uterine tubes) and a common *uterus* and a *vagina* which together receive and transport the ova and sperm. *Mammary glands* are also present as accessory reproductive organs. In most mammals, the ovary, uterus and mammary glands undergo cyclical changes in structure and activity in relationship to hormonal changes associated with the menstrual cycle and pregnancy. Micrographs are shown in Figs 14.1 to 14.10.

14.1 OVARIES

The ovaries (Figs 14.1–14.3) are solid organs composed mainly of connective tissue, and are subdivided into an outer zone, the *cortex,* containing *follicles* in various stages of development, and an inner, highly vascularised zone or core, the *medulla,* which connects with the *mesovarium* and attaches the ovary to a fold of peritoneum joined to the wall of the pelvic cavity. The ovary is surrounded by a cuboidal *germinal epithelium* below which there is a layer of dense connective tissue, the *tunica albuginea.* The outer cortex contains large numbers of small or *primary follicles* each of which encloses an immature egg cell or *oöcyte.* Immature germ cells probably do not originate from the so-called 'germinal epithelium' as was once thought but arise elsewhere in the embryo and migrate into the ovary prior to birth.

At sexual maturity, and under the influence of *follicle-stimulating hormone* from the *anterior pituitary* (= pars distalis), some of the primary follicles begin to mature, and one eventually forms a mature or *Graafian follicle* which bulges from the surface of the ovary. This follicle bursts at *ovulation* to release the oöcyte into the fallopian tube. Ovulation is stimulated by a surge of *luteinising hormone* from the anterior pituitary. During maturation of the follicles, their walls secrete *oestrogen* which is responsible for development of the secondary sexual characteristics and the *thickening of the lining of the uterus* (= the endometrium) in preparation for *implantation* of the fertilised ovum (mature oöcyte). The remnants of the

burst follicle in the ovary reorganise under the influence of *prolactin* (also called luteotropin or lactogenic hormone) from the anterior pituitary to form the *corpus luteum* which secretes *progesterone.* This hormone further stimulates the thickening of the uterine wall and influences the development of the secondary sexual characteristics. Unless fertilisation takes place, the corpus luteum degenerates, levels of progesterone and oestrogen fall, and the lining of the uterus breaks down and *menstruation* takes place (*see* Fig. 14.6). If fertilisation occurs, then the corpus luteum continues to secrete progesterone, implantation of the embryo into the uterus occurs, and the *placenta* develops and secretes hormones which *maintain the pregnancy.*

14.2 PLACENTA

The development of the placenta (Figs 14.9 and 14.10) is complex and beyond the scope of this book. Many different types of placenta exist in the mammals, and they have been *classified* in a number of ways, as follows.

(i) *Chorio-vitelline or yolk sac placenta*
This is formed by the connection of the yolk sac with the uterine wall as in marsupials and temporarily in eutherians, e.g. rabbit before the chorio-allantoic placenta takes over (*see* (ii) below).

(ii) *Chorio-allantoic placenta*
This is formed by intimate association of part of the allantois with the chorion and uterine wall. This is most common in higher mammals, e.g. man, in which it is the only method of placentation. In rabbit, it replaces the chorio-vitelline placenta.

(iii) *Chorionic placenta*
This may be a chorio-allantoic placenta or a stage in its development, but may function independently.

Rats, mice, rabbits, guinea pigs, primates, etc., have *chorio-allantoic placentae* which are further classified by the *degree of erosion* of the maternal tissues present and

*See Fig. 3.1 for location of parts.

by the *degree of contact* between foetal and maternal blood (Grosser, 1909, 1927):

(1) *epitheliochorial* — all maternal tissues preserved, e.g. pig;

(2) *syndesmochorial* — uterine epithelium disappears leaving chorion in contact with connective tissue of uterus, e.g. ruminants;

(3) *endotheliochorial* — further reduction of uterine mucosa, e.g. carnivores;

(4) *haemochorial* — complete destruction of uterine tissues so that maternal blood is in direct contact with foetal chorion, e.g. man, rabbit, rat, guinea pig.

The *haemochorial type* (Figs 14.9 and 14.10) is further subdivided into *labyrinthine haemochorial* as in rodents and rabbits, and *villous* as in man. These two types are distinguished by the presence of either trophoblastic tubules (lamellae), in which the maternal blood spaces are small, or by villi (= man) carrying foetal capillaries which are bathed in a large reservoir of maternal blood.

REFERENCES

Grosser, O. (1909). *Eihäute und der Placenta,* Wien and Leipzig.

Grosser, O. (1927). *Frühentwicklung, Eihautbildung und Placentation des Menschen und der Säugetiere*, Bergmann, Munchen.

Parkes, A. S. (ed.) (1958). *Marshall's 'Physiology of Reproduction'*, vol. 2, 3rd edn, Longmans Green, London, New York and Toronto.

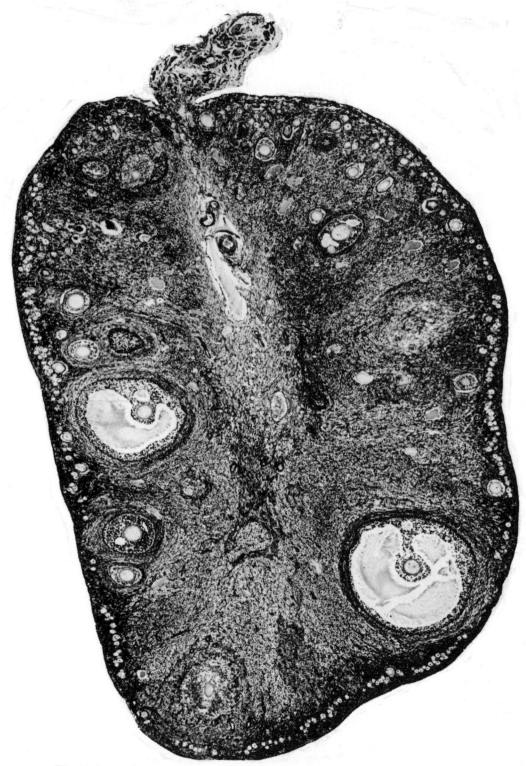

Fig. 14.1.(a) Ovary section (rabbit), low power, Masson's triple stain. ×50

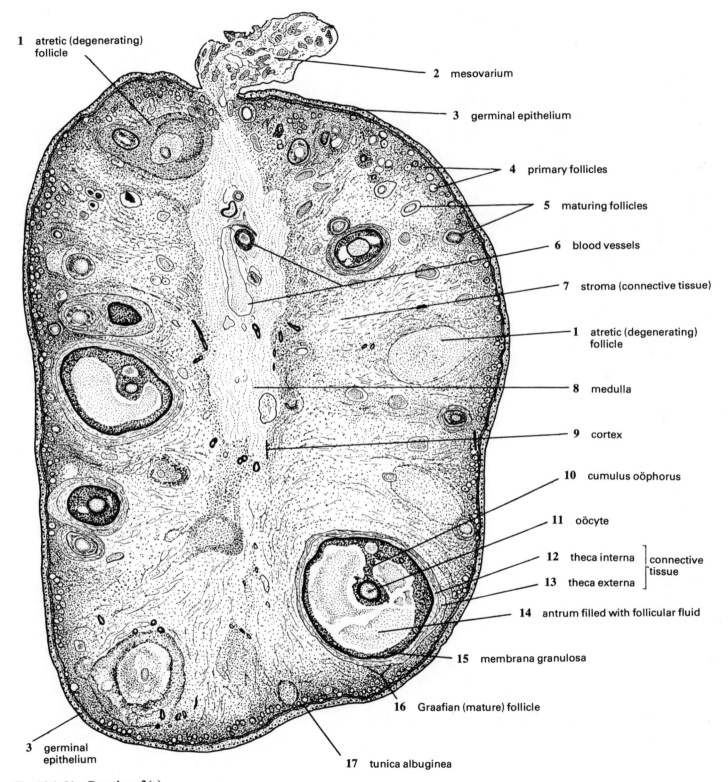

1 atretic (degenerating) follicle

2 mesovarium

3 germinal epithelium

4 primary follicles

5 maturing follicles

6 blood vessels

7 stroma (connective tissue)

1 atretic (degenerating) follicle

8 medulla

9 cortex

10 cumulus oöphorus

11 oöcyte

12 theca interna ⎤ connective
13 theca externa ⎦ tissue

14 antrum filled with follicular fluid

15 membrana granulosa

16 Graafian (mature) follicle

3 germinal epithelium

17 tunica albuginea

Fig. 14.1.(b)   Drawing of (a)

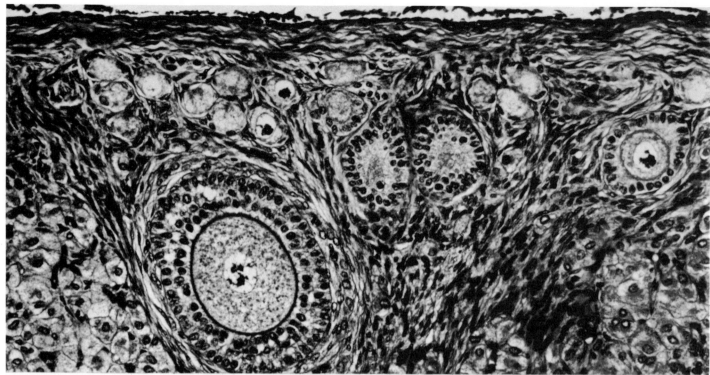

Fig. 14.2.(a)   Ovary section (rabbit), medium power of outer cortex. ×350

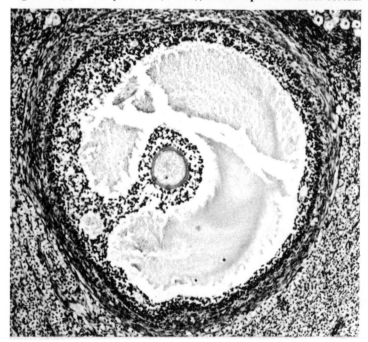

**Fig. 14.2.(b)   Ovary section (rabbit), medium power of
Graafian follicle. ×110**

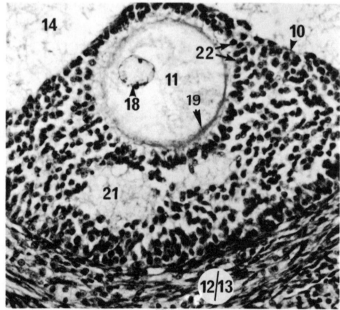

**Fig. 14.2.(c)   Oöcyte (11) (rabbit) in cumulus oöphorus (10) of
Graafian follicle, medium power. Note antrum
(14), thecae interna and externa (12/13), nucleus of
oöcyte (18), zona pellucida (19), Call–Exner vacuole
(21) (accumulation of deeply staining follicular fluid)
and follicle cells forming corona radiata (22). ×280**

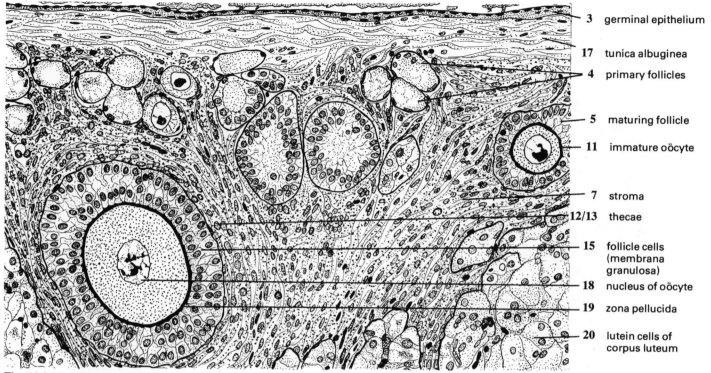

3 germinal epithelium

17 tunica albuginea

4 primary follicles

5 maturing follicle

11 immature oöcyte

7 stroma

12/13 thecae

15 follicle cells (membrana granulosa)

18 nucleus of oöcyte

19 zona pellucida

20 lutein cells of corpus luteum

Fig. 14.2.(d) Drawing of (a)

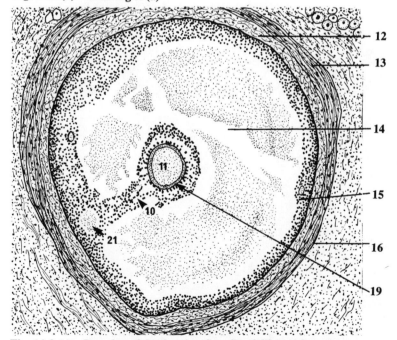

12

13

14

15

16

19

Characteristic features of ovary

(A) Circular outline, solid organ with no lumen

(B) Divided into outer cortex containing many circular follicles of different sizes, and inner fibrous medulla containing blood vessels

(C) Higher power identifies large egg cell (oöcyte) in follicles, connective tissue stroma between follicles and outer, single-layered germinal epithelium

Functions

(A) Produces oöcytes

(B) Cells of membrana granulosa and theca of Graafian follicle synthesise oestrogen (= sex hormone which effects changes in secondary sex organs and causes proliferation of endometrium of uterus)

(C) Corpus luteum secretes progesterone (= sex hormone, stimulates endometrium and prepares it for implantation of fertilised ovum)

Fig. 14.2.(e) Drawing of (b) showing Graafian follicle (16), antrum with follicular fluid (14), cumulus oöphorus (10), oöcyte (11), thecae interna (12) and externa (13), membrana granulosa (15), zona pellucida (19), Call–Exner vacuole (21)

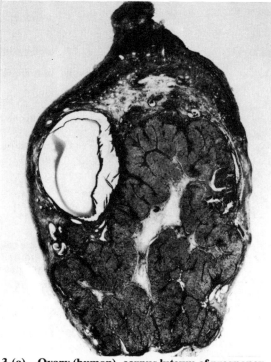

Fig. 14.3.(a) Ovary (human), corpus luteum of pregnancy, low-power section. ×6

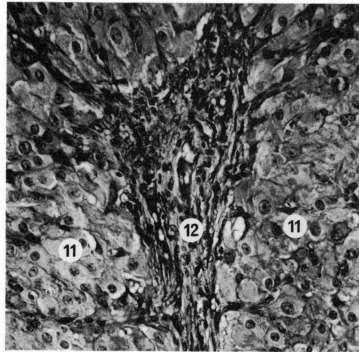

Fig. 14.3.(b) Ovary (human), corpus luteum, high power showing two cell types in wall — the granulosa lutein cells (11) and less common, more deeply staining theca lutein cells (12). ×280

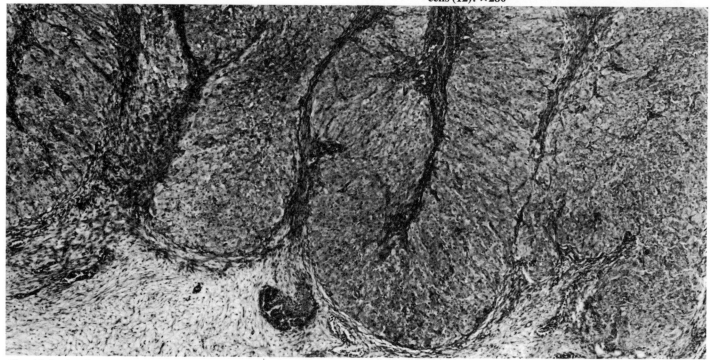

Fig. 14.3.(c) Ovary (human), corpus luteum, medium power. Note highly folded nature of glandular tissue forming wall. ×60

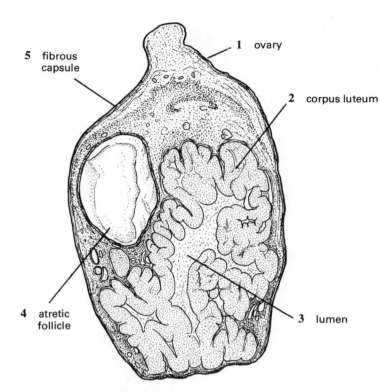

5 fibrous capsule

1 ovary

2 corpus luteum

4 atretic follicle

3 lumen

Fig. 14.3.(d)   Drawing of (a)

Characteristic features of corpus luteum

(A)   One only usually present in humans (several in other mammals, e.g. rat) and fills up to 50% of ovary

(B)   Wall much infolded and composed mainly of typical light-staining endocrine secretory cells (= granulosa lutein cells) very similar to those of the islets of Langerhans

(C)   Centres of infoldings are darker staining and composed of connective tissue and theca lutein cells

Functions

(A)   Secretes oestrogen which suppresses follicle stimulating hormone from pituitary

(B)   Secretes progesterone which builds up endometrium of uterus to receive fertilised ovum and form placenta

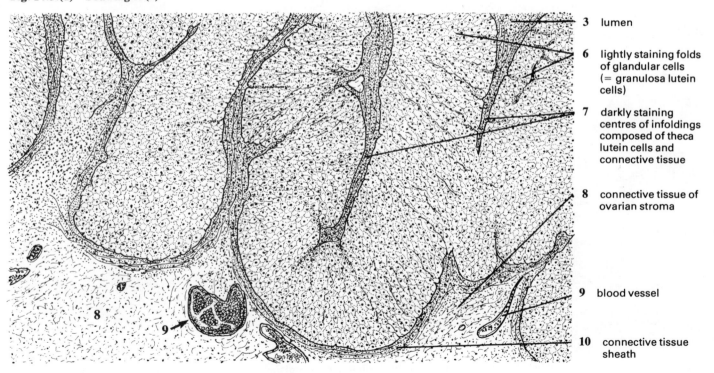

3   lumen

6   lightly staining folds of glandular cells (= granulosa lutein cells)

7   darkly staining centres of infoldings composed of theca lutein cells and connective tissue

8   connective tissue of ovarian stroma

9   blood vessel

10   connective tissue sheath

Fig. 14.3.(e)   Drawing of (c)

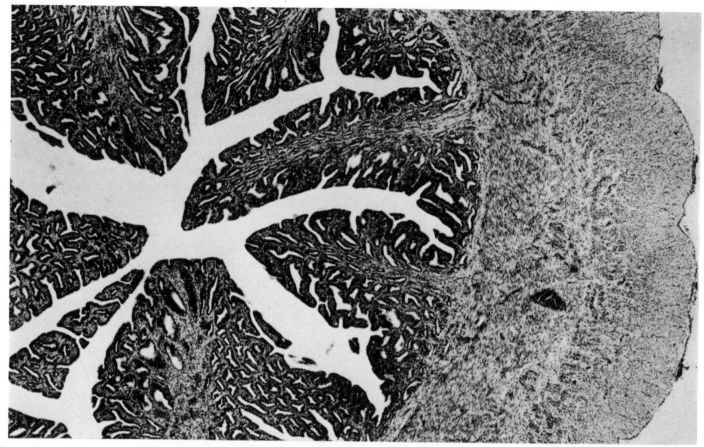

Fig. 14.4.(a)   Fallopian tube (= oviduct or uterine tube) (rabbit), low power, T.S. ×55

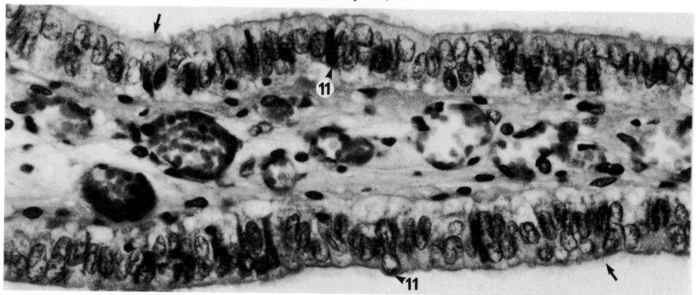

Fig. 14.4.(b)   Fallopian tube (rabbit), high power of mucosa. Note ciliated cells (unlabelled arrows) and secretory cells (11) (= peg cells). ×750

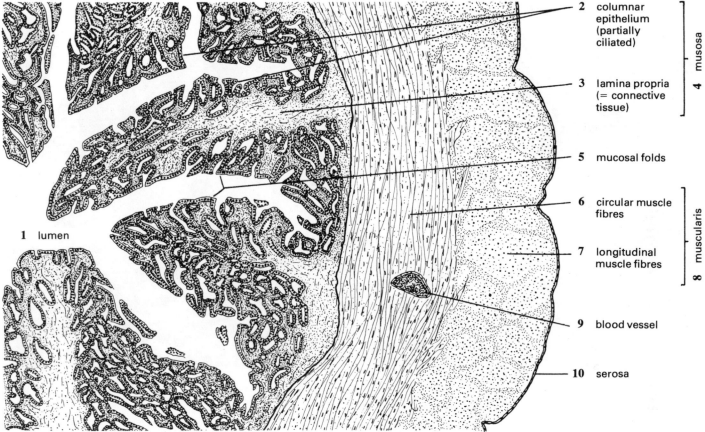

1 lumen

2 columnar epithelium (partially ciliated)

3 lamina propria (= connective tissue)

4 musosa

5 mucosal folds

6 circular muscle fibres

7 longitudinal muscle fibres

8 muscularis

9 blood vessel

10 serosa

Fig. 14.4.(c)   Drawing of (a)

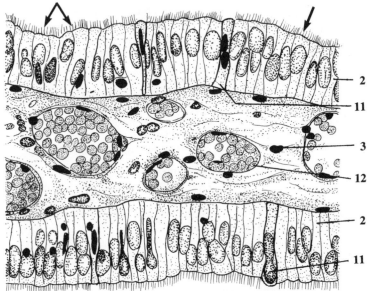

2

11

3

12

2

11

Fig. 14.4.(d)   Drawing of (b). Note ciliated cells (unlabelled arrows) and secretory cells (= peg cells) (11), fibroblasts of connective tissue (3) and capillaries (12)

Characteristic features of fallopian tube

(A)   Superficially resembles gut but, in contrast, epithelium is partially ciliated and no submucosa or glands present

(B)   Muscular coat not divided into well-defined longitudinal and circular layers

(C)   Lumen extremely restricted by large mucosal folds

Functions

(A)   Conveys ova from ovaries to uterus

(B)   Site of fertilisation of ovum by sperm

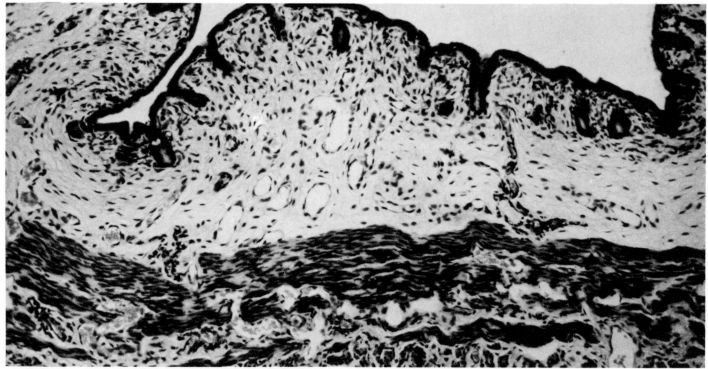

Fig. 14.5.(a)   Uterus (rabbit), low power, T.S. ×80

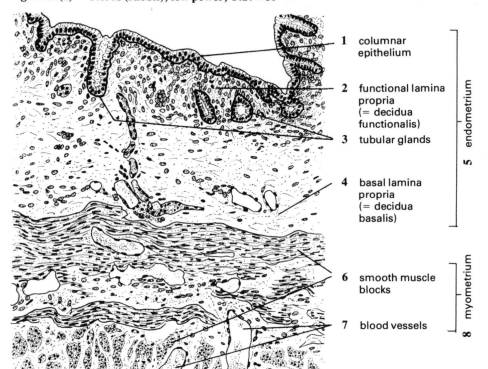

Fig. 14.5.(b)   Drawing of right-hand side of (a)

1 columnar epithelium

2 functional lamina propria (= decidua functionalis)

3 tubular glands

4 basal lamina propria (= decidua basalis)

5 endometrium

6 smooth muscle blocks

7 blood vessels

8 myometrium

Characteristic features of uterus

(A)   Variable morphology depending on stage of female reproductive cycle

(B)   Thick lamina propria (endometrium) contains tubular or coiled glands = invaginations of surface epithelium

(C)   Unlike gut, tubular glands widely spaced, no submucosa present and muscular coat not divided into well defined layers

(D)   Only limited folding of lining

Functions

(A)   Endometrium forms site of implantation of fertilised ovum (= blastocyst) and site of formation of placenta

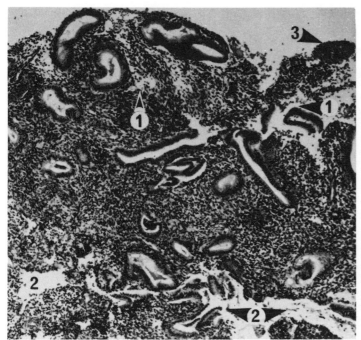

Fig. 14.6.(a) Uterus (human), low-power section during menstrual phase. Note sloughing off of outer endometrium (1), loss of epithelium, damaged glands (2) and blood clots (3). ×85

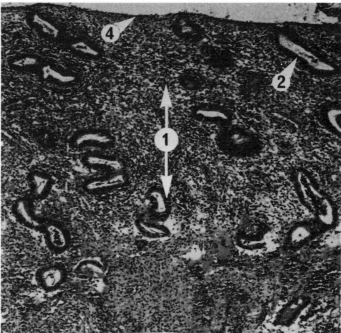

Fig. 14.6.(b) Uterus (human), low-power section during proliferative (= follicular, oestrogenic or reparative) phase. Note reappearance of columnar epithelium (4) and tubular, often straight, glands (2) in reformed outer endometrium (1). × 80

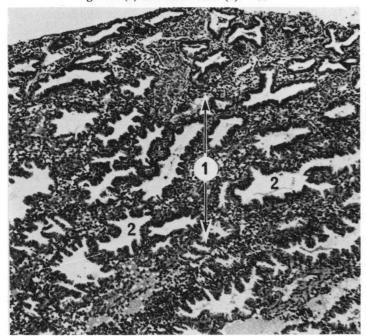

Fig. 14.6.(c) Uterus (human), low-power section during secretory (= progravid or progestational) phase. Note highly developed, corkscrew-shaped glands (2) in thickened outer endometrium (1). ×85

Uterine cycle

In primates, a well-marked female reproductive cycle exists which in humans takes approximately 28 days. This represents the number of days between each menstrual flow. During the menstrual phase (days 1—4) (Fig. 14.6 (a)), neither oestrogen from mature follicles nor progesterone from the corpus luteum are present in high enough concentration to maintain the outer endometrium which is sloughed off. As a follicle matures in the ovary, so oestrogen concentration increases and the outer endometrium regenerates during the proliferative phase (days 5—14) (Fig. 14.6 (b)). Ovulation occurs (day 14), a corpus luteum forms and secretes progesterone, and the endometrium is further stimulated and the glands activated during the secretory phase (Fig. 14.6 (c)). Fertilisation and pregnancy cause retention of corpus luteum but normally this shrinks at approximately day 24, progesterone levels fall and the outer endometrium is shed (= menstrual phase) (Fig. 14.6 (a)) and a new cycle begins.

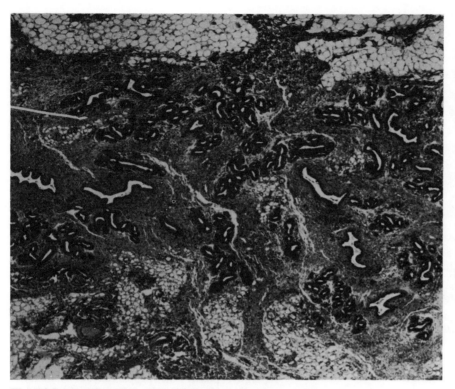

Fig. 14.7.(a)   Mammary gland, inactive, low power, section. ×60

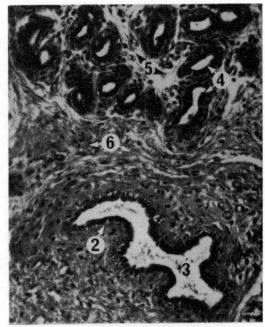

Fig. 14.7.(b)   **Mammary gland, inactive, medium power of part of a lobule showing stratified cuboidal epithelium (2) lining the duct (3) and tubules (4). Note also intralobular (5) and interlobular (6) connective tissue. Section. ×250**

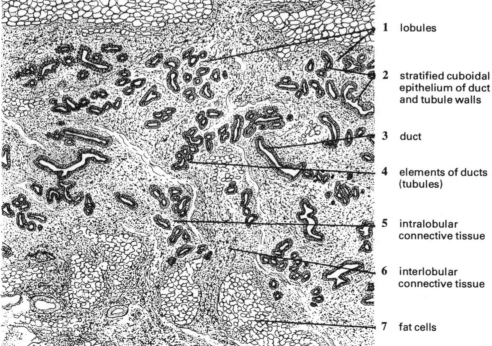

Fig. 14.7.(c)   **Drawing of (a)**

1 lobules

2 stratified cuboidal epithelium of duct and tubule walls

3 duct

4 elements of ducts (tubules)

5 intralobular connective tissue

6 interlobular connective tissue

7 fat cells

Characteristic features of inactive mammary gland

(A)   Resembles sweat glands in skin (*see* Chapter 9) although ducts usually larger and the secretory portion of sweat glands is lined by columnar and not stratified cuboidal epithelium

(B)   Composed of numerous lobules containing tubular elements

(C)   Lobules contain and are surrounded by masses of connective tissue, fat is also often present between lobules

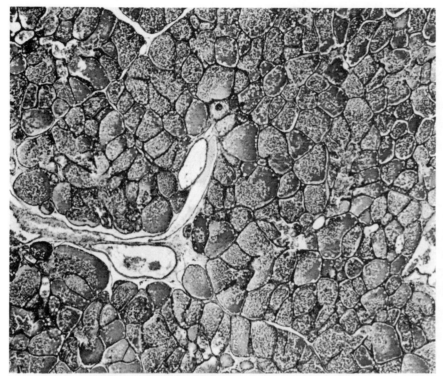

Fig. 14.8.(a)   Mammary gland, lactating, low power, section. ×60

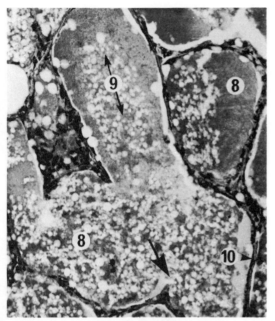

Fig.14.8.(b)   Mammary gland, lactating, medium power showing simple cuboidal epithelium (10), lining alveoli (8). Note interconnecting alveoli (unlabelled arrow) and secretory products (9). Section. ×250

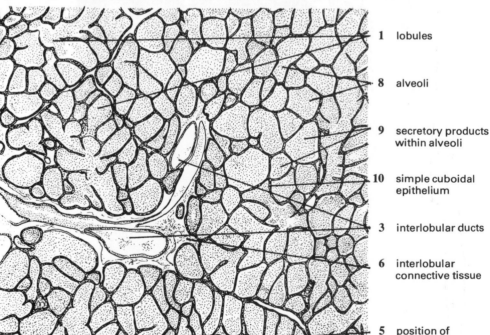

1	lobules
8	alveoli
9	secretory products within alveoli
10	simple cuboidal epithelium
3	interlobular ducts
6	interlobular connective tissue
5	position of intralobular connective tissue

Fig. 14.8.(c)   Drawing of (a)

Characteristic features of lactating mammary gland

(A)   Resembles thyroid gland (*see* Chapter 15) but can be distinguished by interconnection of some alveoli

(B)   Numerous alveoli formed by proliferation from ducts and lined by cuboidal epithelium

(C)   Alveoli filled with secretory product containing fat droplets which are usually extracted during processing to leave many small holes

(D)   Ducts present and alveoli arranged in lobules

Functions

Alveoli produce milk for nutrition of young, in first few days after birth. This secretion is rich in colostrum which contains antibodies for protection of newborn from infection. Milk is ejected by means of the milk ejection reflex elicited by suckling young and stimulated by oxytocin release from posterior pituitary

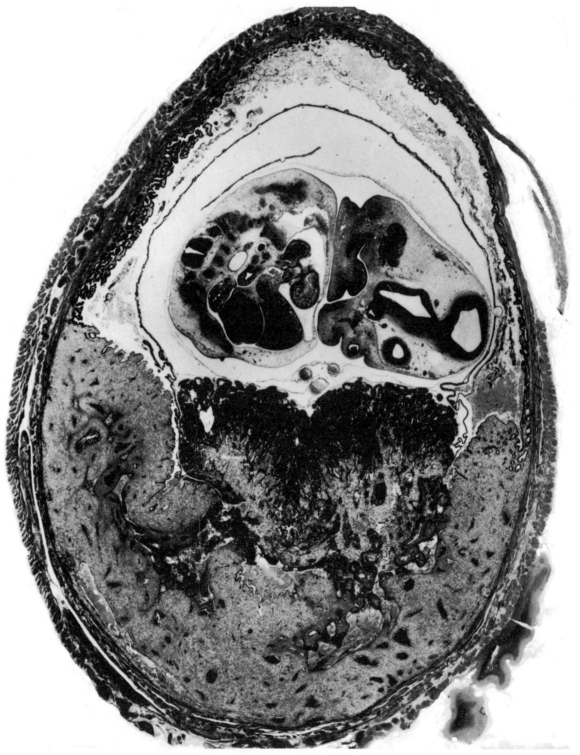

Fig. 14.9.(a)   Uterus (rabbit), section during the second half of pregnancy showing placenta and developing embryo. Low power,
Masson's triple stain. ×10

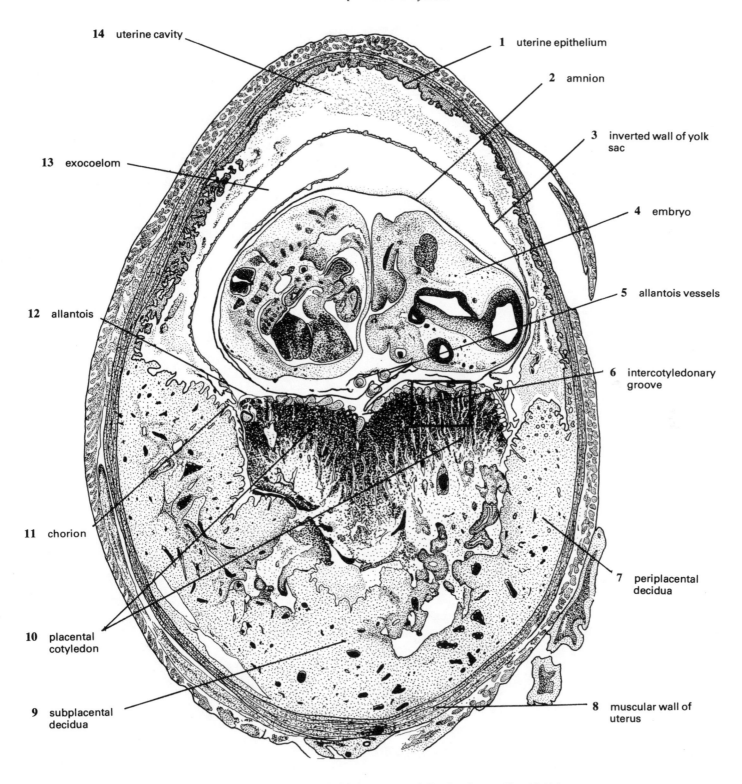

14 uterine cavity

1 uterine epithelium

2 amnion

3 inverted wall of yolk sac

13 exocoelom

4 embryo

5 allantois vessels

12 allantois

6 intercotyledonary groove

11 chorion

7 periplacental decidua

10 placental cotyledon

8 muscular wall of uterus

9 subplacental decidua

Fig. 14.9.(b) Drawing of (a). ×9. *N.B.* Boxed area is shown in high power on following figure (Fig. 14.10.)

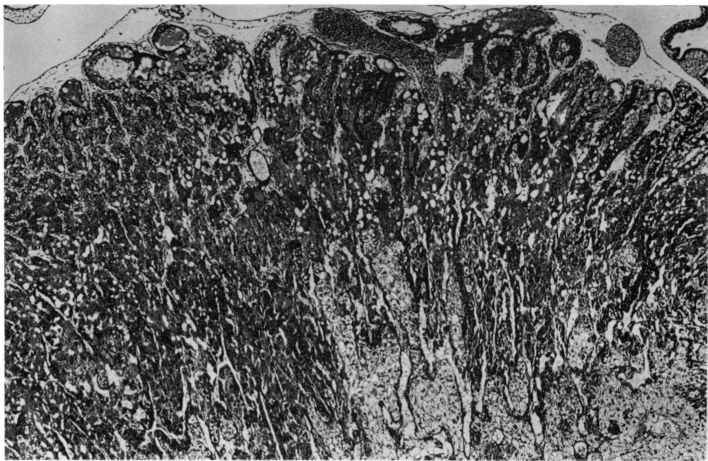

Fig. 14.10.(a) Placenta (rabbit), low power of boxed region of Fig. 14.9b, showing numerous trophoblastic tubules separating the foetal and maternal blood. Masson's triple stain. ×60

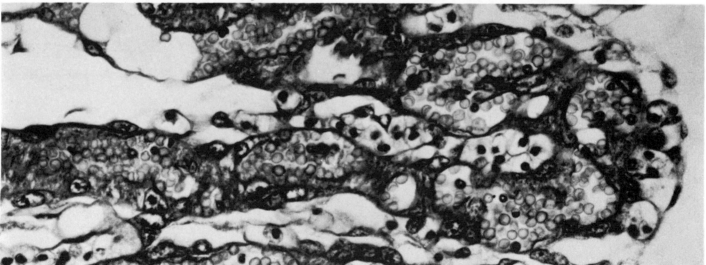

Fig. 14.10.(b) Placenta (rabbit), high power of boxed region in (c) showing apex of trophoblastic tubule. Note foetal and maternal erythrocytes separated by thin membranes. Masson's triple stain. ×625

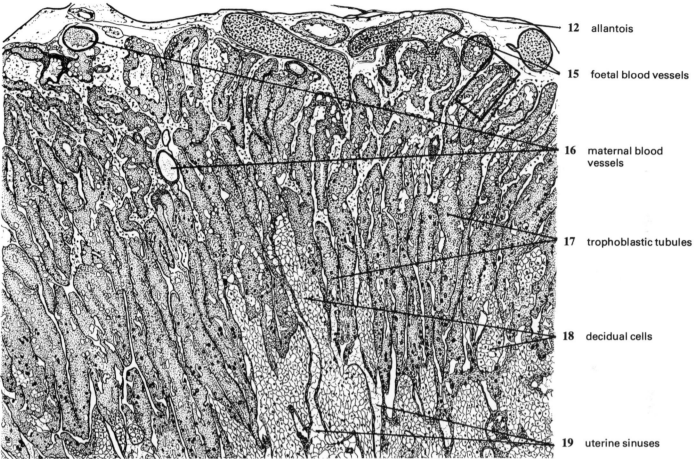

12 allantois

15 foetal blood vessels

16 maternal blood vessels

17 trophoblastic tubules

18 decidual cells

19 uterine sinuses

Fig. 14.10.(c) **Drawing of (a) showing numerous trophoblastic tubules (17) separating the foetal (15) and maternal (16) blood**

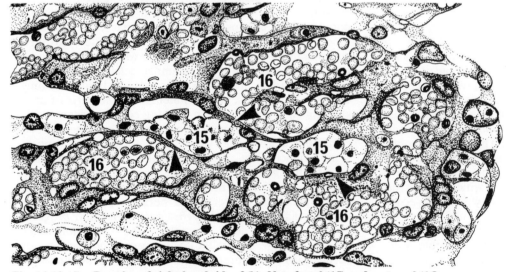

Fig. 14.10.(d) **Drawing of right-hand side of (b). Note foetal (15) and maternal (16) erythrocytes separated by thin membranes (arrowheads)**

Characteristic features of placenta

(A) Contains numerous hollow tubules (in rabbit) or villi (in man) bathed and filled by blood

(B) Appears rather disorganised and unlike gut, etc., not clearly divided into distinct layers

(C) Usually intimately associated with uterus and embryo

Functions

(A) Carries oxygen, food, etc., to developing embryo and removes foetal waste products

(B) Secretes oestrogen, progesterone and gonadotrophic hormones which maintain pregnancy to term

15 Endocrine Organs*

As mentioned in Chapter 4, endocrine glands have lost their connections (or ducts) to the outer surface of the body and discharge their products directly into the bloodstream. They are thus also termed *ductless glands* and their secretions are called *hormones*. Hormones are *chemical messengers* in the body and affect many aspects of cellular physiology and behaviour.

The main endocrine organs (micrographs are shown in Figs 15.2 to 15.8) are the *pituitary,* a pair of *adrenal glands,* the *thyroid,* four (or fewer in some animals, e.g. rat only has two) *parathyroids* and the *pineal body.* Endocrine activity, however, is also associated with the pancreas, testes, ovaries, placenta, kidneys and digestive system, and also perhaps with the thymus gland. The *pituitary* and *adrenal glands,* because of their complexity, are dealt with in some detail.

15.1 PITUITARY GLAND (= HYPOPHYSIS)

This gland (Figs 15.1 to 15.3) is found just below the base of the brain from which it is partially derived and with which it is connected by a stalk. The pituitary is divided into the *neurohypophysis* (a downgrowth from forebrain) and the *adenohypophysis* (an upgrowth from roof of embryonic mouth). It produces at least *ten hormones* (Fig. 15.1), many of which influence the activity of the other endocrine glands.

The adenohypophysis includes the *pars distalis, pars tuberalis* and *pars intermedia* (*see* Fig. 15.2), but it is the pars distalis, or *anterior lobe* as it is called, which occupies the bulk of the adenohypophysis and the pituitary as a whole. The *pars distalis* is composed of three types of cells, the *acidophils, basophils* and *chromophobes,* named according to their staining reactions. The chromophobes (resistant to staining) probably do not produce specific hormones but may differentiate into the acidophils and basophils. These latter two cell types, which cannot be clearly distinguished using haematoxylin and eosin staining, synthesise particular hormones. Thus the *acidophils* secrete *somatotropin* and *prolactin* (= lactogenic or luteotrophic hormone), while the *basophils* secrete *follicle-stimulating hormone, thyrotropin, adrenocorticotro-*

phic hormone, and *luteinising hormone.* The *pars intermedia* also contains basophilic cells which secrete *melanocyte-stimulating hormone* and the peptide *β-lipotropin* (a precursor molecule).

The *neurohypophysis* includes the *median eminence* which links the brain with the second and third parts of the neurohypophysis, the *infundibular stalk* and the *pars nervosa.* The neurohypophysis is really an extension of the brain and is composed of *nerve fibres* and cells supposedly related to neuroglia (= supporting cells of the nervous system), the *pituicytes.* Two hormones are associated with the neurohypophysis, *oxytocin* and *vasopressin* (otherwise known as antidiuretic hormone). It now seems likely that oxytocin and vasopressin are actually synthesised in the *hypothalamus* of the forebrain and are merely stored in the neurohypophysis.

15.2 ADRENAL (= SUPRARENAL) GLANDS

These (Figs 15.4 and 15.5) are paired glands usually capping the upper end of each kidney and are divided into *two distinct regions* with different structures and functions. The outer region, the *cortex,* forms the majority of the organ and consists of cords of cells running from the outer capsule to a lighter-staining central region, the *medulla,* composed of clumps of large columnar cells and small blood vessels. The cortex is usually subdivided into three zones: a thin outer *zona glomerulosa* which is composed of darkly staining groups of columnar cells, a thick middle *zona fasciculata* made up of cords of lighter-staining, empty-looking cells, and an inner *zona reticularis* of dark-staining cells arranged as branching cords adjacent to the medulla. The zona glomerulosa secretes the *mineralocorticoids* (e.g. *aldosterone)* which regulate sodium and potassium balance. The zona fasciculata and zona reticularis secrete the *glucocorticoids* (e.g. *cortisol, corticosterone,* etc.) which affect carbohydrate metabolism and have an anti-inflammatory effect, and perhaps certain sex hormones such as the *androgens, oestrogens* and *progesterone.* The medulla secretes the *catecholamines, epinephrine* (= adrenaline) and *norepinephrine* (= noradrenaline) which prepare the body for stress conditions

*See Fig. 3.1 for location of various organs.

(i.e. 'fight or flight'). The release of the glucocorticoids of the adrenal cortex is mainly regulated by *adrenocortico-* *trophic hormone* (ACTH) from the anterior pituitary (= pars distalis).

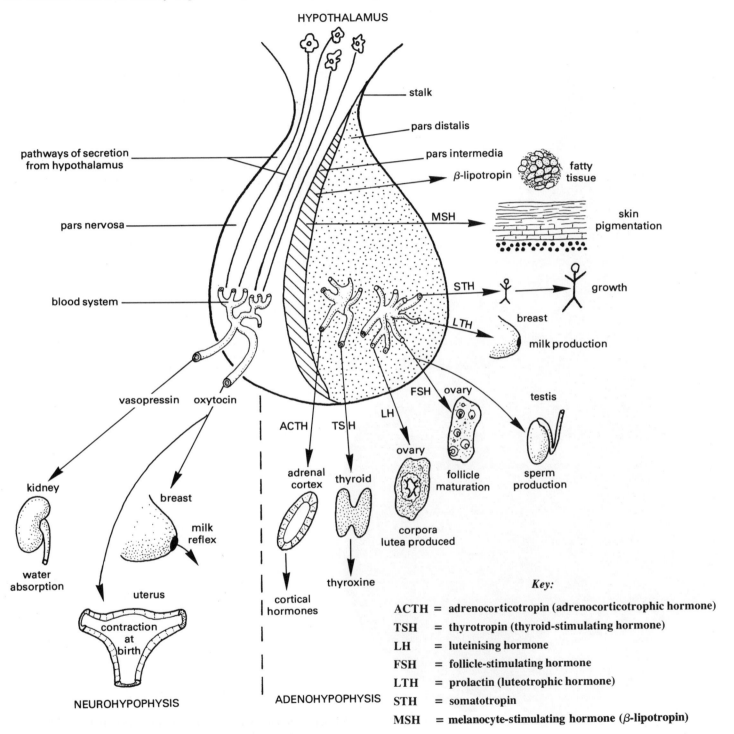

HYPOTHALAMUS

stalk

pars distalis

pars intermedia

pathways of secretion from hypothalamus

β-lipotropin

fatty tissue

MSH

skin pigmentation

pars nervosa

STH

growth

blood system

LTH

breast

milk production

vasopressin   oxytocin

FSH   ovary

testis

ACTH   TSH

LH

kidney

breast

milk reflex

ovary

follicle maturation

sperm production

adrenal cortex

thyroid

corpora lutea produced

water absorption

uterus

contraction at birth

cortical hormones

thyroxine

Key:

NEUROHYPOPHYSIS

ADENOHYPOPHYSIS

ACTH = adrenocorticotropin (adrenocorticotrophic hormone)

TSH = thyrotropin (thyroid-stimulating hormone)

LH = luteinising hormone

FSH = follicle-stimulating hormone

LTH = prolactin (luteotrophic hormone)

STH = somatotropin

MSH = melanocyte-stimulating hormone (β-lipotropin)

Fig. 15.1.   Summary of hormone production by pituitary gland

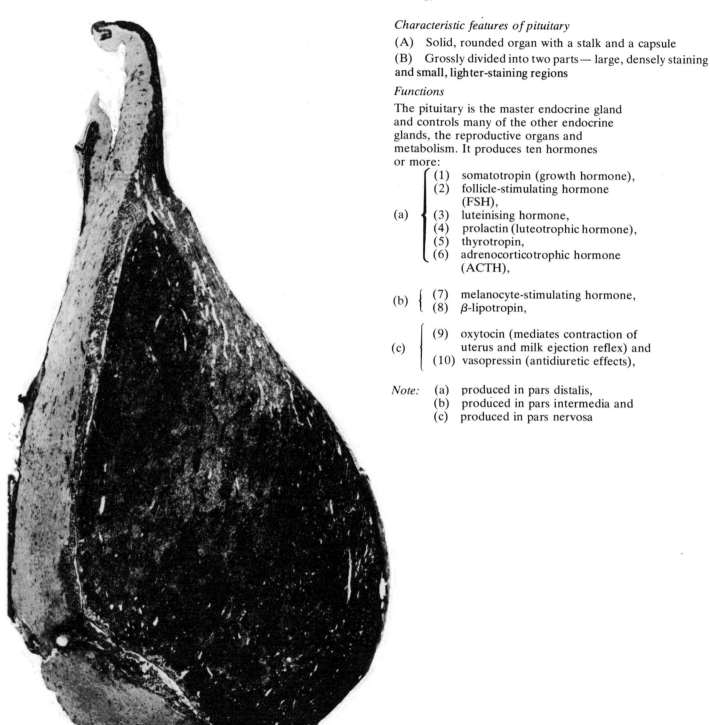

Characteristic features of pituitary

(A) Solid, rounded organ with a stalk and a capsule

(B) Grossly divided into two parts — large, densely staining and small, lighter-staining regions

Functions

The pituitary is the master endocrine gland and controls many of the other endocrine glands, the reproductive organs and metabolism. It produces ten hormones or more:

(a) {
(1) somatotropin (growth hormone),
(2) follicle-stimulating hormone (FSH),
(3) luteinising hormone,
(4) prolactin (luteotrophic hormone),
(5) thyrotropin,
(6) adrenocorticotrophic hormone (ACTH),

(b) {
(7) melanocyte-stimulating hormone,
(8) β-lipotropin,

(c) {
(9) oxytocin (mediates contraction of uterus and milk ejection reflex) and
(10) vasopressin (antidiuretic effects),

Note: (a) produced in pars distalis,
(b) produced in pars intermedia and
(c) produced in pars nervosa

Fig. 15.2.(a)   Pituitary (= hypophysis) (sheep), low power, sagittal (= median longitudinal) section, azan stain. ×14

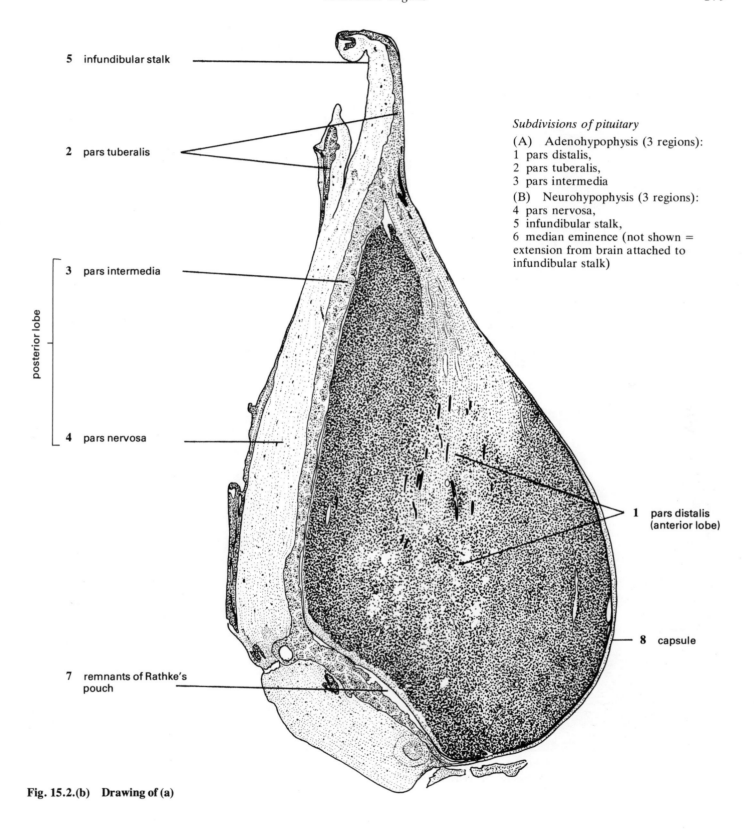

5 infundibular stalk

2 pars tuberalis

Subdivisions of pituitary

(A)   Adenohypophysis (3 regions):
1 pars distalis,
2 pars tuberalis,
3 pars intermedia
(B)   Neurohypophysis (3 regions):
4 pars nervosa,
5 infundibular stalk,
6 median eminence (not shown =
extension from brain attached to
infundibular stalk)

3 pars intermedia

posterior lobe

4 pars nervosa

1 pars distalis
(anterior lobe)

8 capsule

7 remnants of Rathke's
pouch

Fig. 15.2.(b)   Drawing of (a)

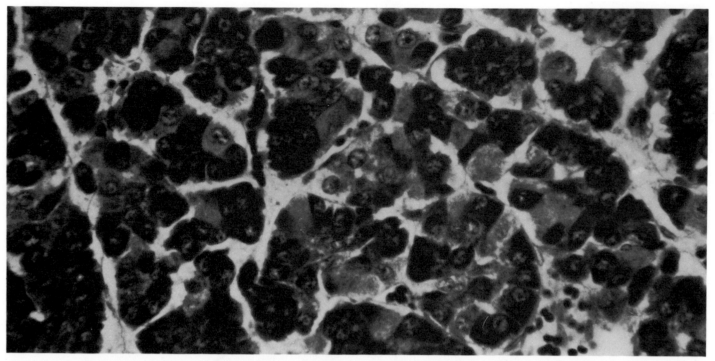

Fig. 15.3.(a)   Pars distalis of pituitary (sheep), high power, section showing chromophilic (= acidophils and basophils) and occasional chromophobic cells. Azan stain. ×750

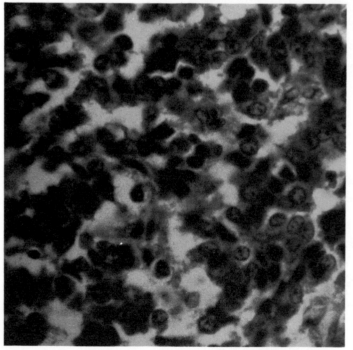

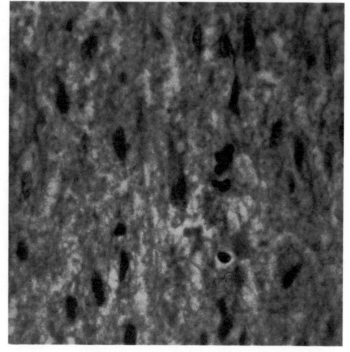

Fig. 15.3.(b)   Pars intermedia of pituitary (sheep), section high power. Note mainly basophilic cells. Azan stain. ×800

Fig. 15.3.(c)   Pars nervosa of pituitary (sheep), section high power. Note nerve fibres and pituicytes. Azan stain. ×750

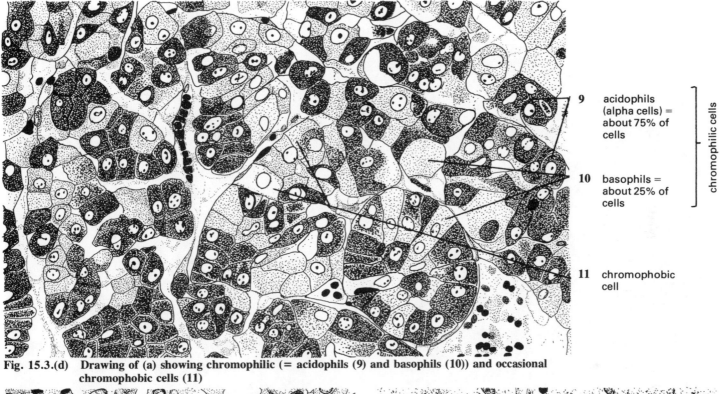

9   acidophils
    (alpha cells) =
    about 75% of
    cells   chromophilic cells

10 basophils =
    about 25% of
    cells

11 chromophobic
    cell

Fig. 15.3.(d)   Drawing of (a) showing chromophilic (= acidophils (9) and basophils (10)) and occasional chromophobic cells (11)

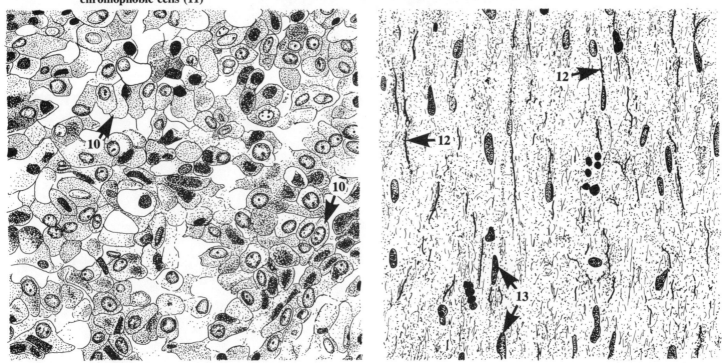

Fig. 15.3.(e)   Drawing of (b). Note mainly basophilic cells (10)

Fig. 15.3.(f)   Drawing of (c). Note nerve fibres (12) and pituicytes (13)

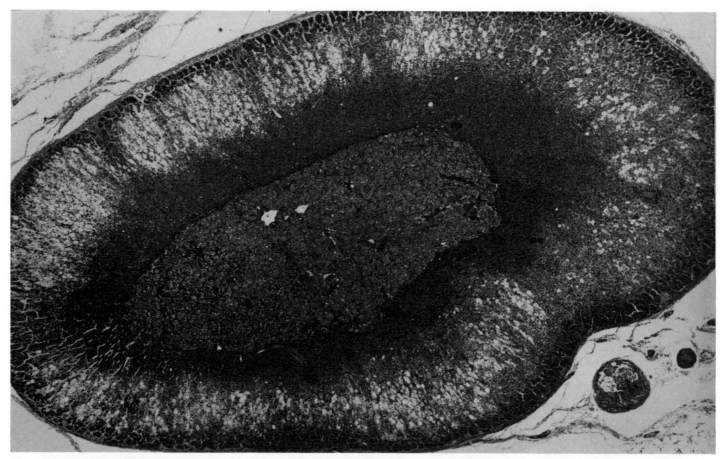

Fig. 15.4.(a)   **Adrenal gland (cat), low-power section, azan stain. ×50**

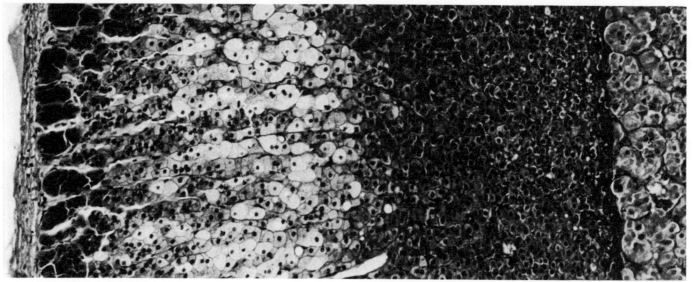

Fig. 15.4.(b)   **Adrenal gland (cat), medium power, section showing general structural and staining characteristics of three cortical zones and medulla. Azan stain. ×230**

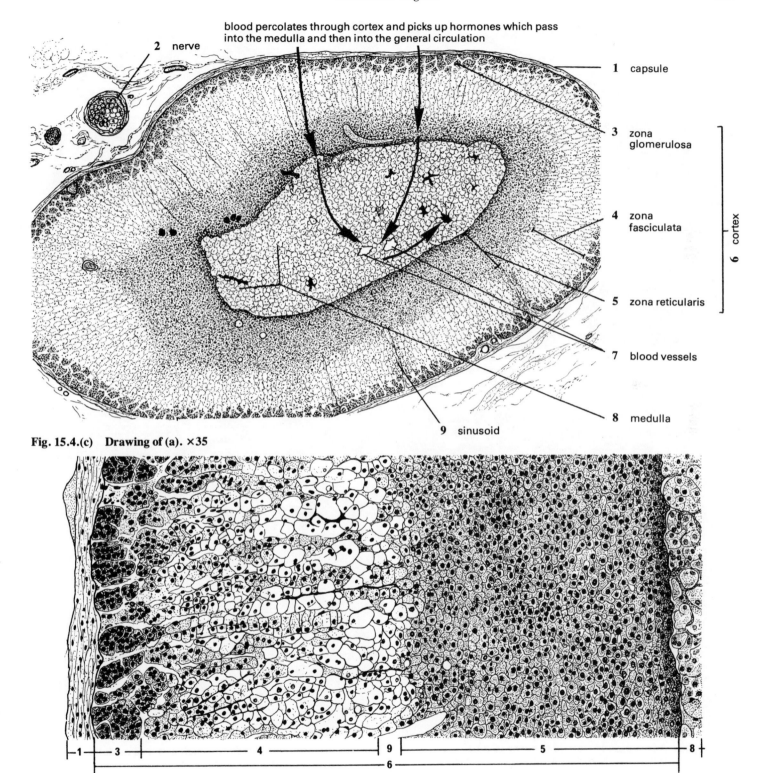

2 nerve

blood percolates through cortex and picks up hormones which pass into the medulla and then into the general circulation

1 capsule

3 zona glomerulosa

4 zona fasciculata

6 cortex

5 zona reticularis

7 blood vessels

8 medulla

9 sinusoid

Fig. 15.4.(c) Drawing of (a). ×35

‑1‑ ‑3‑ ‑4‑ ‑9‑ ‑5‑ ‑8‑

‑6‑

Fig. 15.4.(d) Drawing of (b) showing general structural and staining characteristics of three cortical zones (3, 4, 5) and medulla (8)

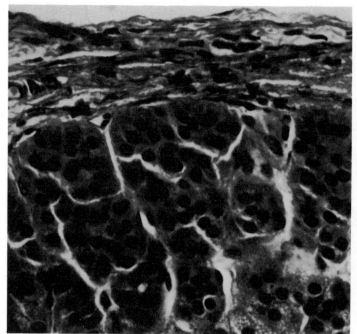

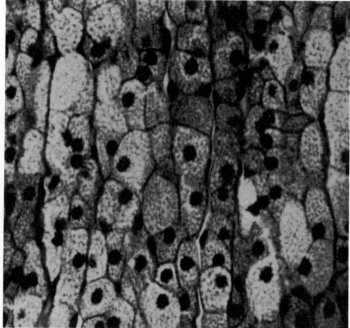

Fig. 15.5.(a)   Adrenal gland (cat), high power showing outer region of cortex. Note fibrous capsule and dark-staining bunches of zona glomerulosa cells. Azan stain. ×650

Fig. 15.5.(b)   Adrenal gland (cat), high power of zona fasciculata. Note light-staining, empty-looking cells arranged in parallel columns. Azan stain. ×650

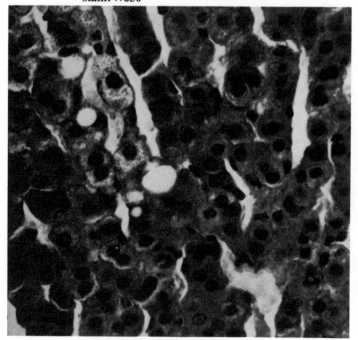

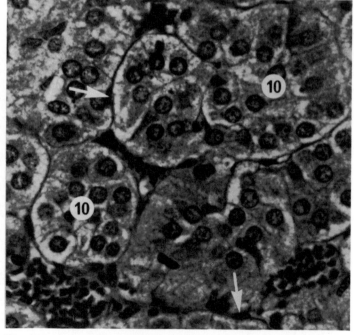

Fig. 15.5.(c)   Adrenal gland (cat), high power of zona reticularis. Note dark-staining, compact cells arranged in branching cords separated by expanded sinusoids. Azan stain. ×650

Fig. 15.5.(d)   Adrenal gland (cat), high power of medulla. Note light-staining, bunches of chromaffin cells (10) and connective tissue cells (arrows). Second cell type (ganglion cells) absent here. ×650

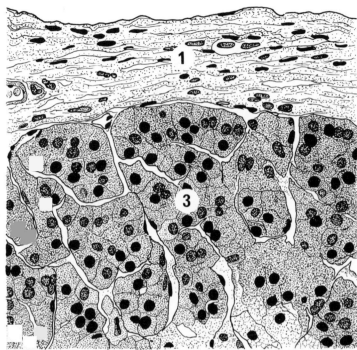

Fig. 15.5.(e)   Drawing of (a). Note fibrous capsule (1) and dark-staining bunches of zona glomerulosa cells (3)

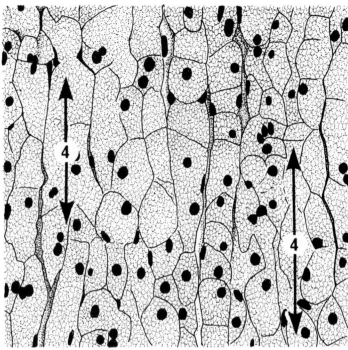

Fig. 15.5.(f)   Drawing of (b). Note light-staining, empty-looking cells arranged in parallel columns (4)

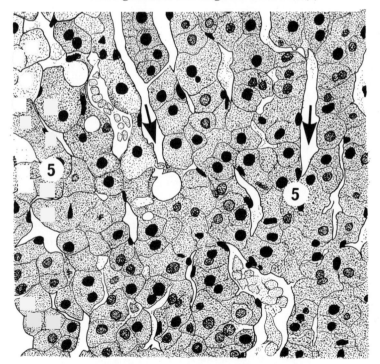

Fig. 15.5.(g)   Drawing of (c). Note dark-staining, compact cells arranged in branching cords (5) separated by expanded sinusoids (arrows)

Characteristic features of adrenal gland

(A)   Solid organ, surrounded by capsule and clearly divided into medulla and cortex

(B)   Unlike kidney, no glomeruli in cortex nor is a ureter present

(C)   Parallel columns of cells form outer region of cortex

(D)   Small bunches of light-staining cells form medulla

Functions

(A)   Cortex secretes three groups of steroid hormones:
(1) mineralocorticoids (e.g. aldosterone) regulate sodium and potassium balance via kidneys,
(2) glucocorticoids (e.g. cortisol) have anti-inflammatory action and affect blood sugar, etc.,
(3) sex hormones supplement those of gonads or have their own specific actions

(B)   Medulla secretes catecholamines (e.g. adrenaline), prepares body for stress conditions ('fight or flight')

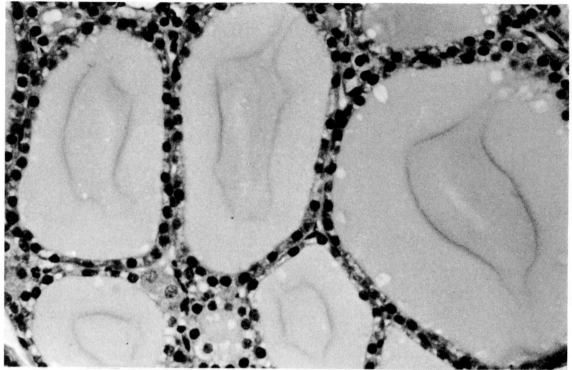

Fig. 15.6.(a) **Thyroid gland (cat); medium power, section. × 500**

Characteristic features of thyroid gland

(A)   Composed of numerous follicles lined by low cuboidal/columnar epithelium; the shape of the cells depends upon the activity of the tissue

(B)   Follicles filled with secretion (colloid)

(C)   Colloid often has scalloped edge at periphery adjacent to epithelium

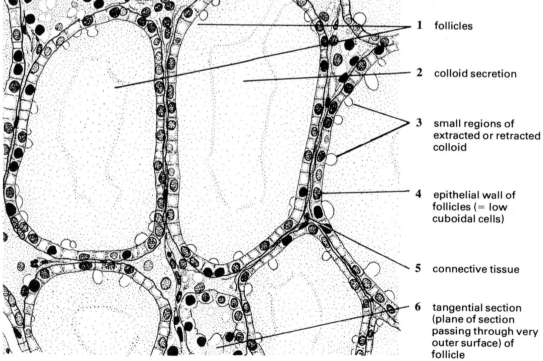

1   follicles

2   colloid secretion

3   small regions of extracted or retracted colloid

4   epithelial wall of follicles (= low cuboidal cells)

5   connective tissue

6   tangential section (plane of section passing through very outer surface) of follicle

Fig. 15.6.(b)   **Drawing of (a)**

Functions

(A)   Most follicle cells secrete the hormones T3 (tri-iodothyronine) and T4 (thyroxine, also called tetra-iodothyronine) which are stored in the colloid. They influence energy metabolism, growth, etc.

(B)   Small numbers of parafollicular cells, which are difficult to find, secrete calcitonin which lowers calcium levels

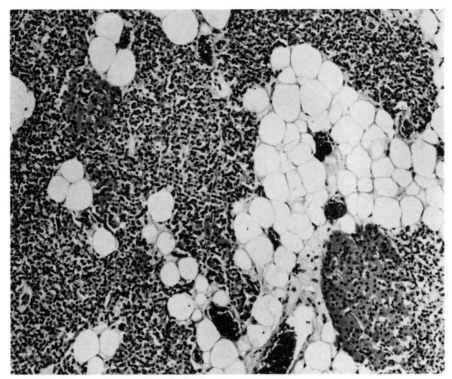

Fig. 15.7.(a)   Parathyroid gland (human), low power, section. ×130

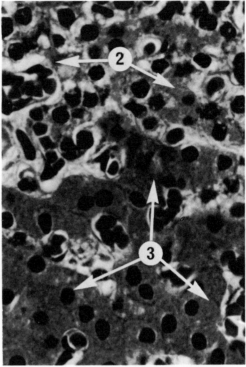

Fig. 15.7.(b)   Parathyroid gland (human).
Note two cell types — chief cells
(2) with islands of oxyphil cells
(3). High power. ×850

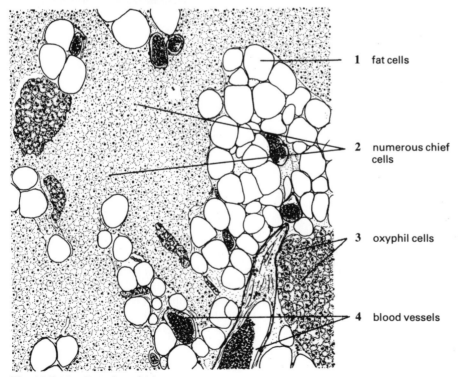

1   fat cells

2   numerous chief
    cells

3   oxyphil cells

4   blood vessels

Fig. 15.7.(c)   Drawing of (a)

Characteristic features of parathyroid gland

(A)   Superficially resembles pancreas and
serous salivary gland, but main cell type (=
chief cells) *not* arranged in small groups or
acini

(B)   Small 'islands' of larger cells present
(= oxyphil cells) but only in adult human
males

(C)   Groups of fat cells often found in
glands from older people

Functions

(A)   Chief cells secrete parathyroid
hormone (parathormone) which elevates
blood calcium levels

(B)   Function of oxyphil cells unknown

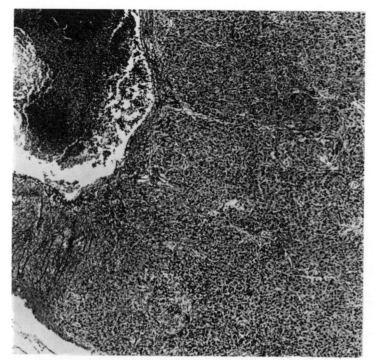

Fig. 15.8.(a) Pineal gland (human), low power, section. ×55

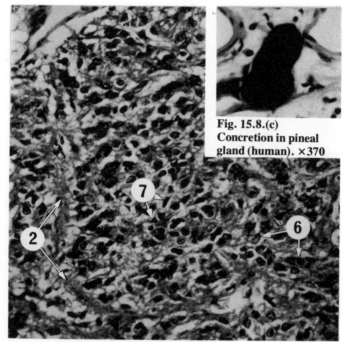

Fig. 15.8.(c)
Concretion in pineal
gland (human). ×370

Fig. 15.8.(b) Lobule of pineal gland (human), high power. Note
two cell types — numerous parenchymal cells (6)
(= pinealocytes) with large nuclei, and glial cells
(7) with smaller elongate nuclei. Trabecula (2).
×280

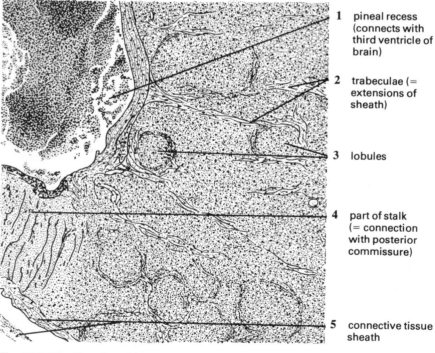

1 pineal recess
   (connects with
   third ventricle of
   brain)

2 trabeculae (=
   extensions of
   sheath)

3 lobules

4 part of stalk
   (= connection
   with posterior
   commissure)

5 connective tissue
   sheath

Fig. 15.8.(d) Drawing of (a)

Characteristic features of pineal gland

(A) Solid gland with connective tissue
sheath and stalk

(B) Divided into lobules by trabeculae
formed of connective tissue

(C) Composed of lightly staining cells
under H.P. (in contrast to lymphoid tissue)
of two types which may be difficult to
differentiate without special staining
techniques

(D) Often contains darkly staining
lamellated deposits = concretions or brain
sand

Functions

(A) Has an antigonadotrophic effect
(delays puberty)

(B) Synthesises melatonin which
modifies skin coloration

(C) Affects renal function

16 Nervous System

Nervous tissue develops from the neural plate of the embryonic ectoderm, and in the adult mammal functions to transmit nervous impulses throughout the animal. Nervous tissue ramifies to practically every part of the body, but forms massive concentrations in certain regions as control centres. These centres are interlinked and together form an integrated whole. The main *subdivisions* of the nervous system are as follows.

(1) The *brain* (Figs 16.3–16.5) and *spinal cord* (Figs 16.6 and 16.7) together form the *central nervous system* — the central coordinating system in the body.

(2) The *peripheral nervous system* serves to communicate the tissues and organs of the body with the central nervous system. It is formed by the *cranial* and *spinal nerves* (e.g. sciatic, Fig. 16.8) and small concentrations of nerve cells or ganglia including the *spinal* (Fig. 16.7) and *sympathetic* (= autonomic) *ganglia*.

(3) A third division of the nervous system called the *autonomic nervous system* contains elements from 1 and 2 and controls the smooth muscles of the viscera and the secretory processes of many of the glands. It is subdivided

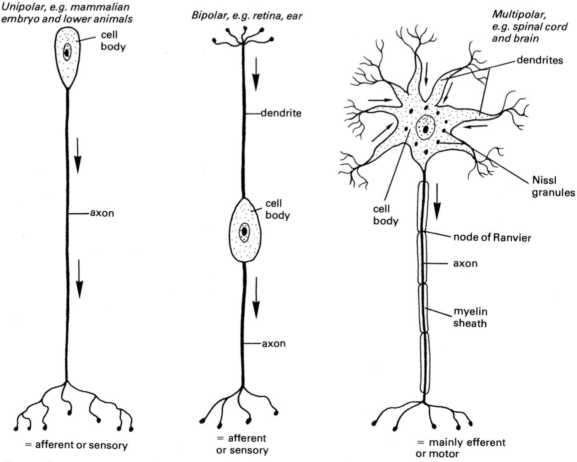

Fig. 16.1 **Types of neurones**

into the *sympathetic* and *parasympathetic* systems, and its activities are usually beyond the control of the conscious mind. The sympathetic system consists of a row of ganglia either side of the nerve cord and associated nerve fibres. It decreases peristalsis, decreases secretion by glands, quickens heart beat, etc. The parasympathetic system consists of nerve fibres and ganglia scattered in the walls of the viscera. It increases peristalsis, increases secretion by glands, slows down heart beat, etc. The autonomic nervous system is only partially under the control of the central nervous system.

16.1 NEURONES

The basic building blocks of the nervous system are the nerve cells, or *neurones,* and associated supporting and connective tissue cells, the *neuroglia.* The neurones (Figs 16.4–16.8) serve to transmit electrical charges or nerve impulses, and structurally they are greatly modified for this function. Each neurone contains a *cell body,* which encloses the nucleus and the cytoplasm with its characteristic *neurofibrils,* and small blocks of basophilic material, or *Nissl bodies.* Unfortunately, the neurofibrils and Nissl bodies only show up satisfactorily after special staining techniques. The neurofibrils can be visualised with silver techniques and appear as delicate threads passing from the cell body into its cytoplasmic extensions (*see* below). The Nissl granules stain well with toluidine blue and represent clumps of ribonucleoprotein involved in protein synthesis. They vary greatly in structure from one type of neurone to another, but are usually very obvious in large motor neurones such as those of the ventral horn of the spinal cord (Fig. 16.6).

Neurones are able to conduct nervous impulses over long distances by means of *cytoplasmic processes (=* nerve fibres), the *dendrites* and the *axons.* These processes are sometimes extremely elongated, and because of them the longest may be up to a metre in length. The dendrite conducts nervous impulses towards the cell body, while the axon conducts the impulses away from the cell body. Nerve fibres usually conduct impulses in one direction only. *Afferent* or *sensory neurones* (from sense organs) transmit impulses towards the central nervous system, while *efferent* or *motor neurones* (to effectors, e.g. muscles, etc.) transmit away from the central nervous system.

Depending upon the number of cytoplasmic processes or nerve fibres, neurones can be classified as *unipolar, bipolar* or *multipolar* (Fig. 16.1).

Unipolar neurones have one process, the axon, and form the afferent (sensory) neurones of many invertebrates. Bipolar neurones have one dendrite and one axon and are also sensory in function. Multipolar neurones have many dendrites and one axon, and are mostly efferent or motor in function, activating skeletal and smooth muscle, glands, etc.

The nerve fibres of the central nervous system and of the larger peripheral nerves are enclosed by a fatty sheath called the *myelin sheath,* which is formed from specialised cells called *Schwann (= neurilemma) cells.* Where two Schwann cells meet, the myelin sheath is absent and indentations called *nodes of Ranvier* are formed (Figs 16.1, 16.8). Such *nerve fibres* are termed myelinated or medullated and form the *white matter* of the central nervous system while the *cell bodies* form the *grey matter.* Not all nerve fibres are myelinated, and many of the smaller fibres of peripheral nerves lack a myelin sheath, although they are enclosed by Schwann cells. Myelin

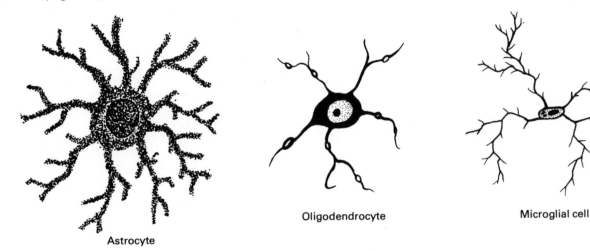

Astrocyte

Oligodendrocyte

Microglial cell

Fig. 16.2. Types of neuroglial cells

sheaths may well increase the speed of transmission of the nerve impulse.

As mentioned above, neurones may be afferent (or sensory) and conduct impulses from the sense organs such as those for smell, sight, hearing, taste, pain, temperature, etc., to the central nervous system, or they may be efferent (or motor) and transmit messages from the central nervous system to muscles, glands, etc. The neurones link up with each other at *synapses* and, although there is no cytoplasmic connection in a synapse, the message is conveyed across the gap of the synapse by a *chemical transmitter*, e.g. *acetylcholine*.

16.2   NEUROGLIA

There are more neuroglial (Figs 16.2 and 16.4) or suppor-tive cells than neurones in the central nervous system. Although termed 'supportive', they do not provide much structural rigidity and may have other functions. There are a number of neuroglial cell types, including the *astrocytes, oligodendrocytes, microglial cells* and *ependymal cells* (Fig. 16.2). The astrocytes are star-shaped, and some of their cytoplasmic extensions expand to form foot plates which surround the blood vessels in the brain and may well control the interchanges that occur between the blood and the interstitial fluid of the brain. The oligoden-drocytes are very like astrocytes, but with fewer processes, and are associated with the nerve fibres and may well be equivalent to Schwann cells. The microglial cells have smaller cell bodies than astrocytes or oligodendrocytes and few processes with many small extensions. They occur throughout the central nervous system. Ependymal cells line the ventricles of the central nervous system and appear like columnar epithelial cells. Below the *pia mater* (= inner of three connective tissue membranes envelop-ing the central nervous system, the other two being the *dura mater* (= outermost) and the *arachnoid membrane* (Fig. 16.7)), the ependymal cells form an external limiting membrane around the central nervous system.

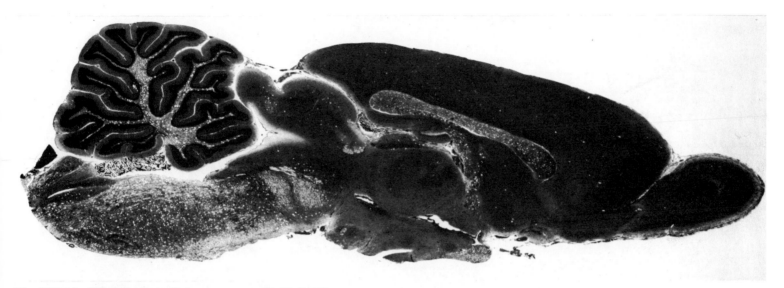

Fig. 16.3.(a)   Whole brain (rat), low power, vertical L.S. ×8

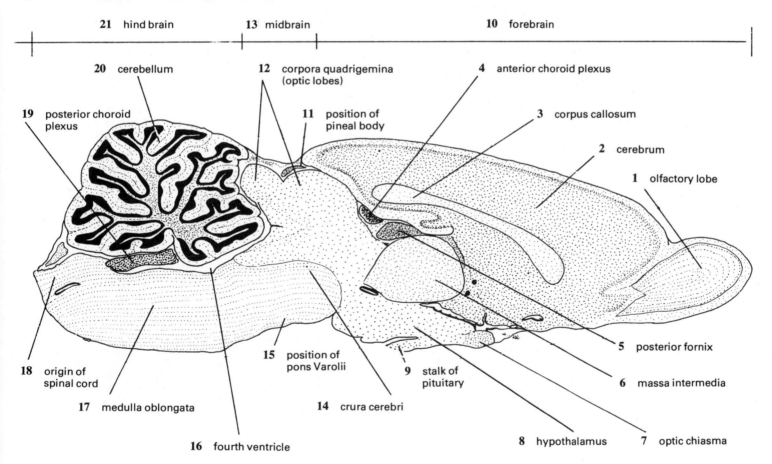

| 21 | hind brain | 13 | midbrain | 10 | forebrain |

20   cerebellum

12   corpora quadrigemina
     (optic lobes)

4   anterior choroid plexus

19   posterior choroid
     plexus

11   position of
     pineal body

3   corpus callosum

2   cerebrum

1   olfactory lobe

5   posterior fornix

18   origin of
     spinal cord

15   position of
     pons Varolii

9   stalk of
    pituitary

6   massa intermedia

17   medulla oblongata

14   crura cerebri

16   fourth ventricle

8   hypothalamus   7   optic chiasma

Fig. 16.3.(b)   Drawing of (a)

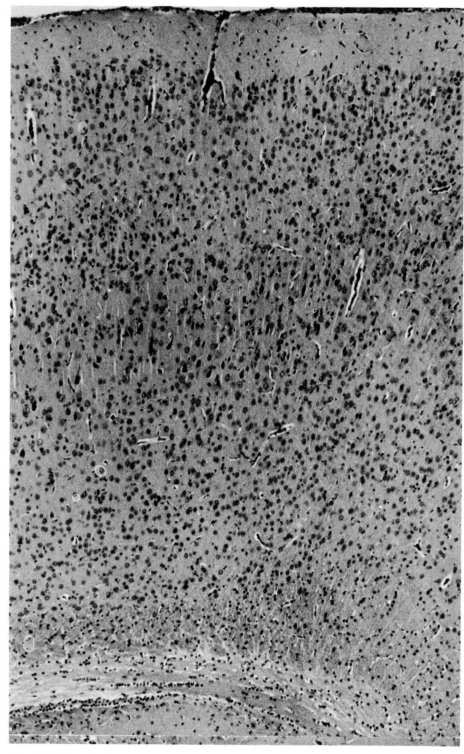

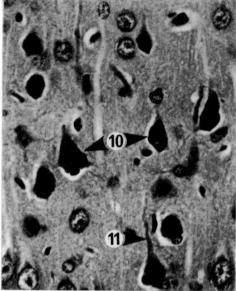

Fig. 16.4.(b) Cerebrum (rat), medium-power section of layer 6 (*see* (d)) stained with haematoxylin and eosin for comparison with section below stained by a silver method. Note large pyramid cells (10) and their dendrites (11) which are not so easy to follow in this H and E preparation. ×450

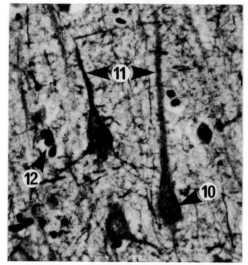

Fig. 16.4.(c) Cerebrum (human), medium-power section of central region showing large pyramidal cells (10) and their dendrites (11). Neuroglial cells (12). Silver stain. ×450

Fig. 16.4.(a)   Cerebrum (rat), low power, section. ×100.
          N.B.   Difficult to distinguish between different layers

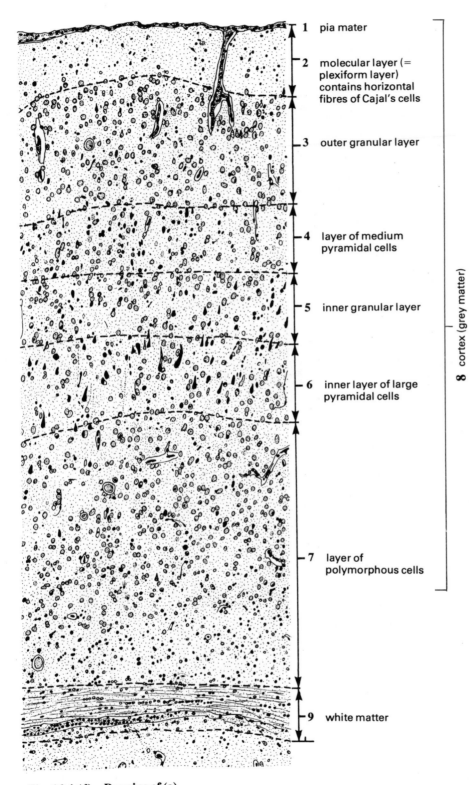

1 pia mater

2 molecular layer (= plexiform layer) contains horizontal fibres of Cajal's cells

3 outer granular layer

4 layer of medium pyramidal cells

5 inner granular layer

6 inner layer of large pyramidal cells

7 layer of polymorphous cells

8 cortex (grey matter)

9 white matter

Fig. 16.4.(d)   Drawing of (a)

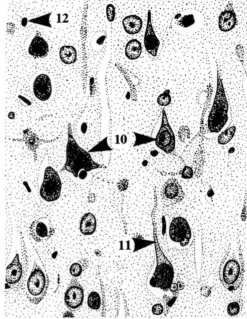

Fig. 16.4.(e)   Drawing of (b) (medium power of layer 6 of (d)). Note large pyramidal cells (10) and their dendrites (11). Neuroglial cells (12)

Characteristic features of cerebrum

(A)   Like all nervous tissue, little or no epithelial, glandular, muscular, lymphoid or connective tissue present and composed of darkly staining cells with fibrous processes

(B)   Surface folded but generally not as much as in cerebellum (Fig. 16.5)

(C)   Cortex not clearly subdivided into various regions with distinct staining properties (compare with cerebellum, Fig. 16.5)

(D)   Pyramidal cells scattered throughout much of cortex

Functions

Multiple, including control of:

(A)   Speech, hearing, smell, touch and sight

(B)   Personality, behaviour and movement

(C)   Memory and perception, etc.

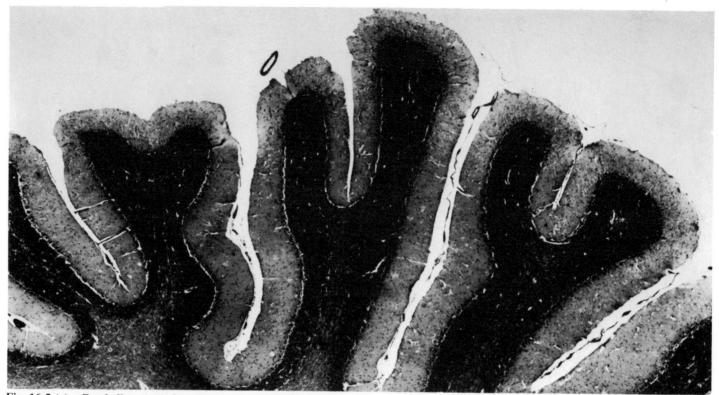

Fig. 16.5.(a)   Cerebellum (cat), low power, section. ×30

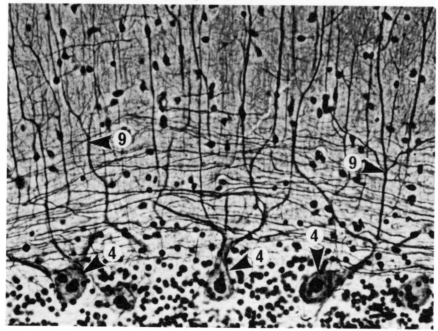

Fig. 16.5.(b)   Cerebellum (human), medium-power section showing Purkinje cells
(4) with their much-branched dendrites (9). Cajal's silver method.
×350

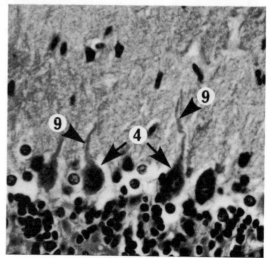

Fig. 16.5.(c)   Cerebellum (human), medium-
power section stained with
haematoxylin and eosin for
comparison with Cajal's stained
section (b). Note that although
Purkinje cells (4) are present, their
dendrites (9) can only be followed
in detail after the special silver
staining. ×450

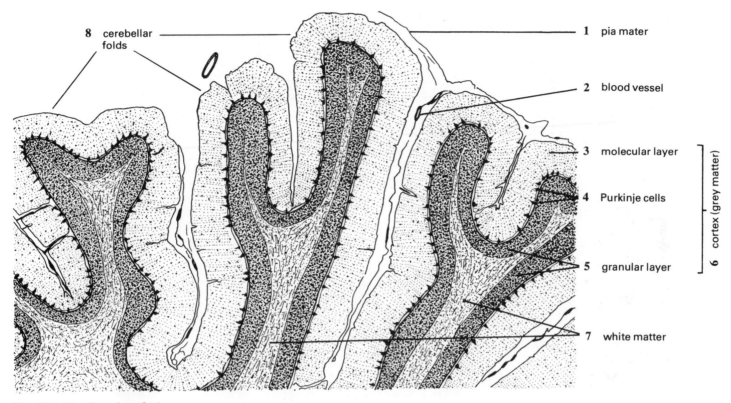

Fig. 16.5.(d) Drawing of (a)

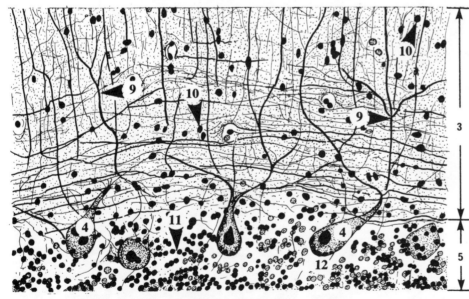

Characteristic features of cerebellum

(A)   Like all nervous tissue, little or no epithelial, glandular, muscular, lymphoid or connective tissues present and composed of darkly staining cells with fibrous processes

(B)   Like cerebrum, the surface is much-folded and a core of lightly staining white matter is present

(C)   Cortex of cerebellum, in contrast to that of cerebrum (Fig. 16.4), is divided into two quite distinct layers — an inner darkly staining granular layer and an outer lighter-staining molecular layer

(D)   Two cortical layers are separated by a layer of giant neurones called Purkinje cells

Functions

(A)   Concerned with coordination of muscular movements

(B)   Also concerned with reflexes which maintain balance and posture

Fig. 16.5.(e) Drawing of (b) showing Purkinje cells (4) with their much-branched dendrites (9). The dendrites ramify the molecular layer (3) which also contains basket cells (10). Note also the granule cells (11) and clear areas (12 = glomeruli) in the granular layer (5)

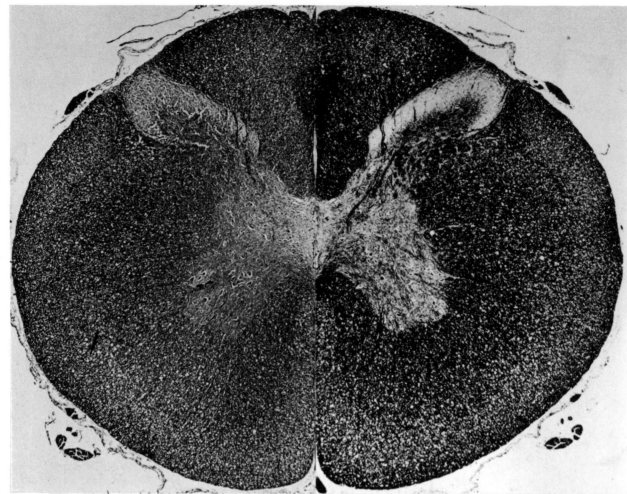

Fig. 16.6.(a) Spinal cord (rabbit), low power, T.S. The figure is a composite of two sections with the left half stained with haematoxylin and eosin (H and E) and the right half by a silver stain. Only the latter stains the nerve fibres clearly. ×40

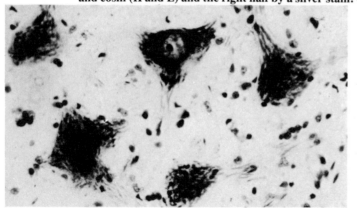

Fig. 16.6.(b) Spinal cord (mammal), medium power of motor neurones in ventral horn of grey matter showing Nissi bodies in cell body, and dendrites. Note also nuclei of neuroglial cells. Toluidine blue. ×300

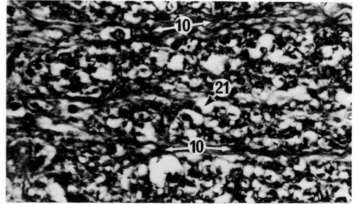

Fig. 16.6.(c) Spinal cord (rabbit), high power showing a portion of the ventral white matter. Note bundles of nerve fibres (10) which form ventral root, and typical myelinated fibres (= axons) (21) in T.S. ×500

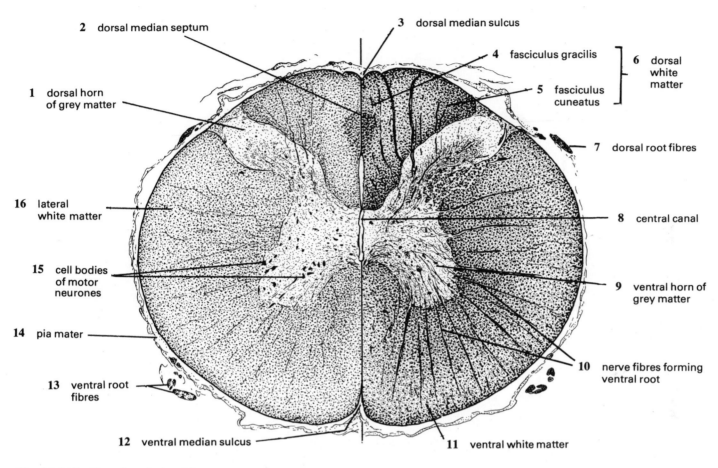

Fig. 16.6.(d)   Drawing of (a). ×30

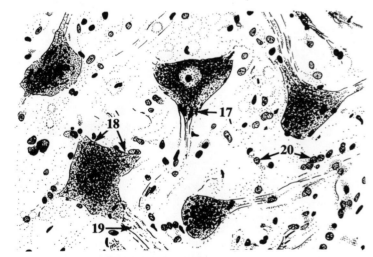

Fig. 16.6.(e)   Drawing of (b) showing Nissl bodies (17) in cell body (18) and dendrites (19). Note also nuclei of neuroglial cells (20)

Characteristic features of spinal cord

(A)   Circular and solid organ with no conspicuous lumen

(B)   Like all nervous tissue, little or no epithelial, glandular, muscular, lymphoid or connective tissues present and composed of cells with fibrous processes

(C)   Most characteristic feature is the central H-shaped grey matter

(D)   Comparatively small in T.S. (Compare cerebrum, medulla, etc.)

Functions

(A)   Supplies nerves to many parts of body and conveys sensory messages to and motor messages from the brain

(B)   Is also responsible for reflex actions and afferent (sensory) and efferent (motor) nerve fibres are directly linked by synapses in grey matter

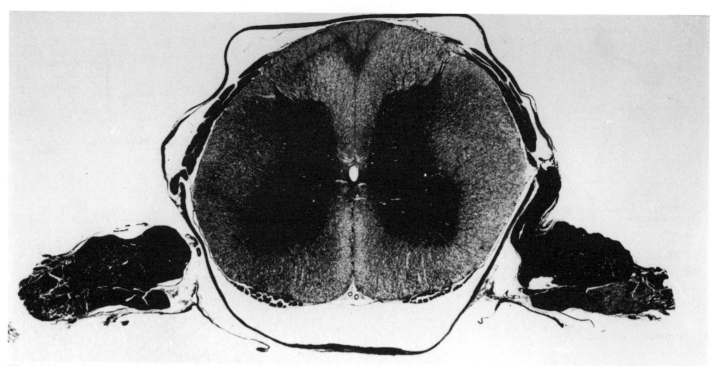

Fig. 16.7.(a)   Spinal cord (mammal), low-power T.S. showing dorsal root ganglion, dorsal root and ventral root fibres. Mallory's staining method. ×12

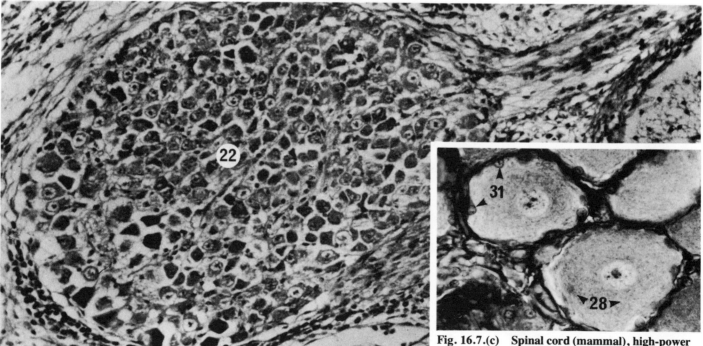

Fig. 16.7.(b)   Spinal cord (rabbit), medium-power section of dorsal root ganglion (22). ×70

Fig. 16.7.(c)   Spinal cord (mammal), high-power section of dorsal root ganglion showing ganglion cells (28) surrounded by satellite cells (31). ×500

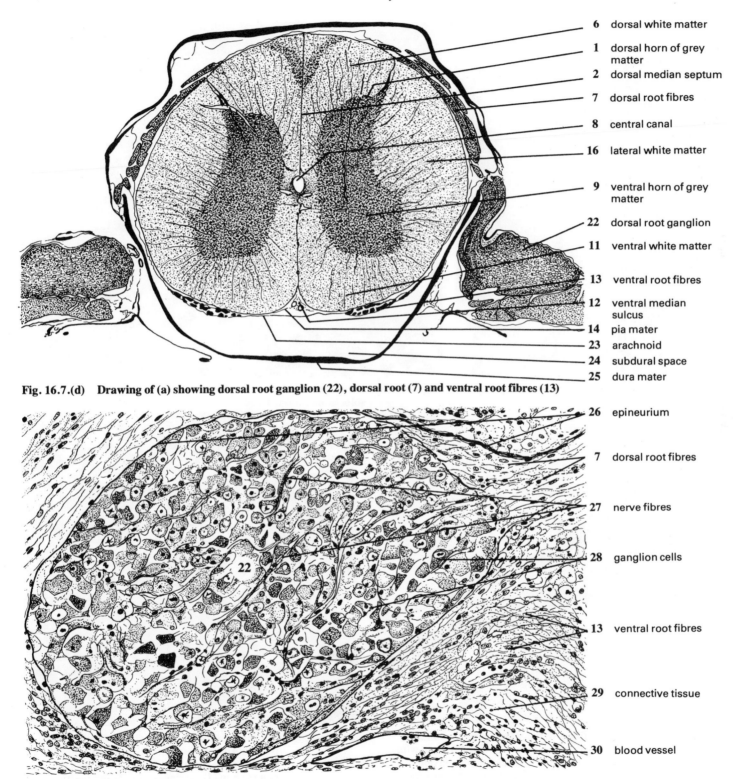

6	dorsal white matter
1	dorsal horn of grey matter
2	dorsal median septum
7	dorsal root fibres
8	central canal
16	lateral white matter
9	ventral horn of grey matter
22	dorsal root ganglion
11	ventral white matter
13	ventral root fibres
12	ventral median sulcus
14	pia mater
23	arachnoid
24	subdural space
25	dura mater

Fig. 16.7.(d)   Drawing of (a) showing dorsal root ganglion (22), dorsal root (7) and ventral root fibres (13)

26	epineurium
7	dorsal root fibres
27	nerve fibres
28	ganglion cells
13	ventral root fibres
29	connective tissue
30	blood vessel

Fig. 16.7.(e)   Drawing of (b)

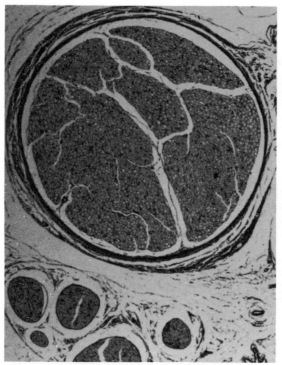

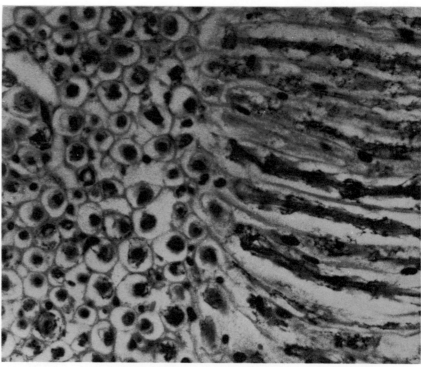

Fig. 16.8.(a)   Nerve (e.g. sciatic, cat), low-power
                 T.S. ×50

Fig. 16.8.(b)   Nerve fibres (sciatic, mammal), high-power section. Acid
                 solochrome stain. ×550

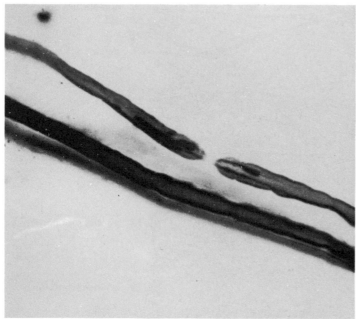

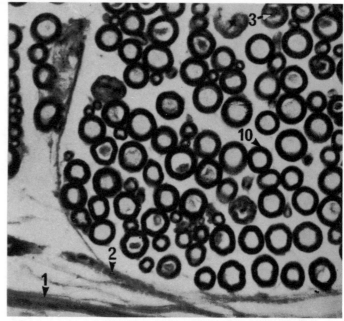

Fig. 16.8.(c)   Whole nerve fibres (from sciatic nerve, mammal),
                 medium power, teased from nerve and treated with
                 osmium tetroxide to show black-staining myelin
                 sheath and node of Ranvier. Axons of nerve fibres
                 also seen. ×400

Fig. 16.8.(d)   Nerve (e.g. sciatic, mammal), medium-power T.S.
                 treated with osmium tetroxide which stains the fat
                 in the myelin sheath (10) black. Note also the
                 epineurium (1), perineurium (2) and position of
                 axons of nerve fibres (3). ×500

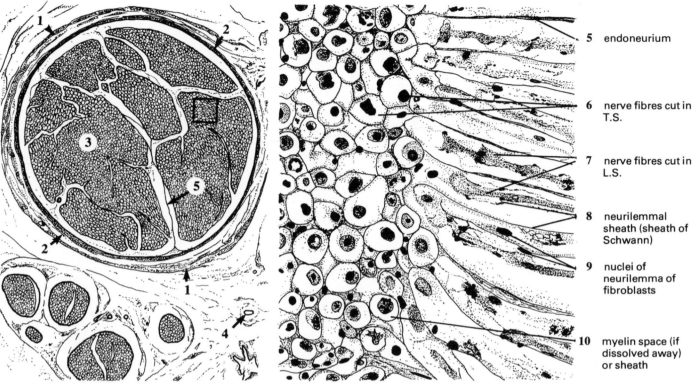

5 endoneurium

6 nerve fibres cut in T.S.

7 nerve fibres cut in L.S.

8 neurilemmal sheath (sheath of Schwann)

9 nuclei of neurilemma of fibroblasts

10 myelin space (if dissolved away) or sheath

Fig. 16.8.(e) Drawing of (a). Note epineurium (1), perineurium (2), bundles of nerve fibres (3), blood vessels (4) and endoneurium (5)

Fig. 16.8.(f) Drawing of (b). High power of region such as that boxed in (e)

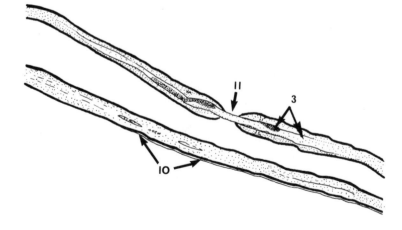

Characteristic features of nerves

(A) Composed of numerous parallel fibres usually arranged in bundles

(B) Bundles of fibres ensheathed in connective tissue

(C) No lumen and little or no epithelial, glandular, muscular or lymphoid tissues present

Functions

Transmits electrical messages to and from brain and spinal cord

Fig. 16.8.(g) Drawing of (c) showing black-staining myelin sheath (10) and node of Ranvier (11). Axons of nerve fibres (3)

17 Sense Organs

Sense organs make an animal aware of what is going on in the internal and external environments. The *nerve fibres* from the cranial and spinal organs end in *receptors* in numerous tissues in the body, and these receptors may be classified as:

interoceptors ⎫
proprioceptors ⎬ all served by *afferent neurones*.
exteroceptors ⎭

17.1 INTEROCEPTORS

These include *deep-seated receptors* that serve the viscera and blood vessels. Good examples of interoceptors are found in the carotid body of the internal carotid artery and the aortic bodies in the aorta. They are *chemoreceptors* and respond to changes in the carbon dioxide and oxygen tensions of the blood. The end result of their activities is to regulate respiration and blood flow according to the needs of the body.

17.2 PROPRIOCEPTORS

These are found in the labyrinth of the inner ear, in the muscles, tendons and joints, and are responsible for the sense of *balance* and *orientation* of the body in relation to its surroundings. A particularly good example of a proprioceptor is provided by the *membranous labyrinth* of the *inner ear*. This consists of not only the *cochlear duct*, which contains the receptors for hearing, but also the three *semicircular canals*, the *utricle* and the *saccule*, which contain the receptors for balance and orientation of the head. Each semicircular canal contains a swelling, the *ampulla*, and this encloses a gelatinous structure, the *cupula*, which moves and stimulates the receptor cells as a result of movements of the head which activate the fluid (the *endolymph*) in the canals. The utricle and the saccule contain similar receptors.

The onion-like *Pacinian corpuscles* are also proprioceptors and are found in the deep layers of the skin (*see* Fig. 9.2), around the viscera, in the connective tissue near joints and tendons, in the pancreas, etc. They are formed of concentric layers of connective tissue penetrated by a large nerve fibre which ends in the centre of the corpuscle. They are concerned with *pressure reception*.

17.3 EXTEROCEPTORS

These include a whole range of receptors which are stimulated by the *external environment*. They include receptors of pain, touch, temperature, smell, taste, sight and sound. The animal is very much aware of the messages received by the exteroceptors.

17.3.1 Pain

Pain is perceived by a network of *naked nerve endings* which arise from many small myelinated and non-myelinated afferent neurones. These nerve endings are extremely widespread in the body and are found throughout the *stratum germinativum* in the epidermis of the skin, in many connective tissues, the viscera, the cornea of the eye, the teeth, etc.

17.3.2 Touch

Tactile receptors are found in the skin and include not only naked nerve endings wrapped around the roots of the

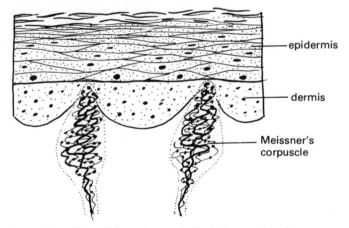

Fig. 17.1. Two Meissner's corpuscles below epidermis

205

hair follicle but also more specialised receptors termed *Merkel's discs* and *Meissner's corpuscles*. Merkel's discs, like the naked nerve endings, perceive light touch and are found, for example, in the tongue. Meissner's corpuscles are more specialised and are encapsulated and composed of a complex of connective tissue cells and nerve endings (Figs 9.2 and 17.1). They occur just below the epidermis especially in the palm side of the fingers and lower surface of the toes.

17.3.3   Temperature

The receptors for heat and cold have not been clearly defined but may involve the mushroom-shaped *corpuscles of Ruffini* and the *end bulbs of Krause,* respectively. They are both found associated with the skin and are encapsulated.

17.3.4   Smell

The receptors for smell (Fig. 17.2) are found scattered between the columnar cells of the *olfactory epithelium* in the highest part of the nose. The sensory cells are *bipolar neurones* with the apex of the cell formed from a modified dendrite which projects above the surface of the epithelium to form the ciliated *olfactory vesicle*. The non-myelinated axon of the neurone penetrates the underlying connective tissue and joins with adjacent fibres to form small olfactory nerve bundles. The surface of the epithelium is kept moist by secretions of special glands, the *Bowman's glands* (not to be confused with the Bowman's capsules in the kidney), and odours dissolve in this fluid, and thus become concentrated and stimulate the receptor cells. Nerve impulses then pass along the olfactory nerve to the olfactory centres of the *cerebrum.*

17.3.5   Taste

Taste receptors, like the receptors of smell, are *chemoreceptors* and are found mainly embedded in the *stratified squamous epithelium* of the *tongue* (*see* Fig. 11.5). They are, however, also found scattered in the pharynx, epiglottis and larynx. The receptors consist of small groups of spindle-shaped *supporting cells* and *sensory cells* which open onto the surface of the epithelium by a small *taste pore*. Each sensory cell receives stimuli through a short taste hair. Substances in solution, e.g. in saliva, enter the taste pores and stimulate the sensory cells from which afferent fibres pass to the *medulla oblongata* and *cerebrum* via the lingual, facial and glossopharyngeal nerves.

17.3.6   Sight

The receptors for sight (Figs 17.3–17.5) are found within the *retina* of the eye. The retina contains *three layers of neurones:* the outermost (i.e. towards the outer surface of the eye) is composed of the *rods* and *cones,* the middle contains the *bipolar cells,* and the innermost is formed by the *ganglion cells* (Fig. 17.4). The rods and cones are the only light-sensitive part of the retina, and the terms 'rod'

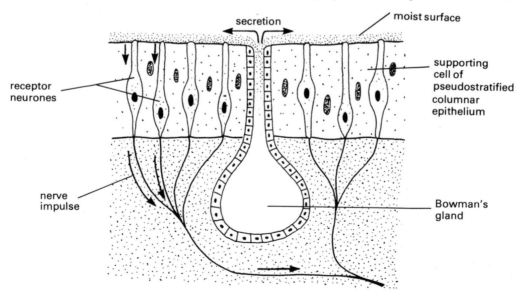

Fig. 17.2.   Part of olfactory epithelium showing receptor cells

and 'cone' refer to the shape of the dendrites emerging from the neurones in this layer. The rods and cones point towards the *pigmented epithelium* which lies just below the fibrous covering of the eye, formed by the *sclera* and *choroid*. The axons of the rod and cone cells pass to the middle part of the retina and synapse with the dendrites of the bipolar cells. The axons of the bipolar cells, in turn, synapse with the dendrites of the innermost layer of neurones, the ganglion cells (Fig. 17.4). The axons of the ganglion cells pass over the inner surface of the retina and at the back of the eye, in the *blind spot,* penetrate the retina and fibrous coat and unite to form the *optic nerve* which travels to the visual area of the *cerebral cortex.* Thus, to reach the photosensitive rods and cones, light rays first have to pass through two non-sensitive layers of neurones in the retina. The rods are sensitive to dim light, while bright light stimulates the cones, which also register colour.

17.3.7 Sound

The receptor organ for hearing (Figs 17.6–17.7) is found in the *cochlea,* which is located in the membranous labyrinth of the *inner ear.* The cochlea is a bony structure containing a spiral tunnel, and is thus like a snail's shell resting on its base. The spiral tunnel is divided longitudinally into three smaller spiral tunnels by two membranes, the *Reissner's* (= vestibular) membrane and, below this, the *basilar membrane.* The middle tunnel, between these two membranes, is the *cochlear duct* (= *scala media*) and this contains the specialised receptor cells for hearing which together form the spiral-shaped *organ of Corti.* This consists of a group of supporting cells in which are embedded special sensory cells, the *hair cells,* which make contact via their apical 'hairs' (= microvilli) with a small shelf called the *tectorial membrane.* The whole organ of Corti rests on the basilar membrane. The afferent fibres from the hair cells make contact with the spiral ganglion in the *modiolus* (= central column of bone) of the cochlea which in turn forms the *cochlear nerve.*

Sound waves are gathered by the *pinna* (= outer ear) and passed to the *tympanic membrane* which vibrates and causes the *auditory ossicles* (= *malleus, incus* and *stapes* = middle ear) to vibrate. The stapes are in contact with the fluid-filled inner ear at the oval window (= *fenestra ovalis*) and transmit the vibrations via the oval window to this fluid (= endolymph in cochlear duct). Vibration of the endolymph results in vibrations of the basilar membrane on which the organ of Corti sits. The hair cells are thus stimulated since they move up and down and tug against the tectorial membrane.

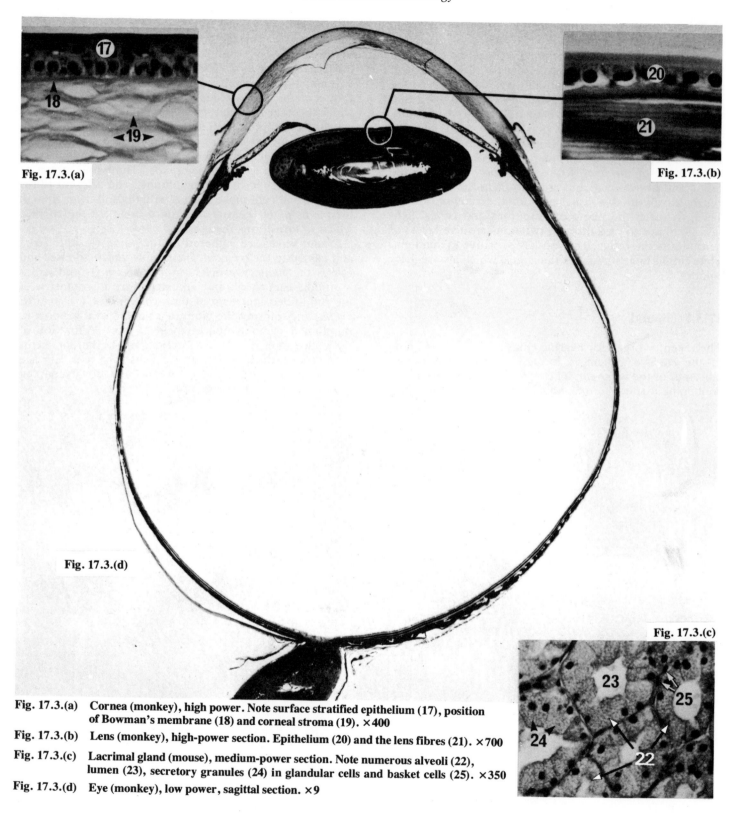

Fig. 17.3.(a)

Fig. 17.3.(b)

Fig. 17.3.(d)

Fig. 17.3.(c)

Fig. 17.3.(a)   Cornea (monkey), high power. Note surface stratified epithelium (17), position of Bowman's membrane (18) and corneal stroma (19). ×400

Fig. 17.3.(b)   Lens (monkey), high-power section. Epithelium (20) and the lens fibres (21). ×700

Fig. 17.3.(c)   Lacrimal gland (mouse), medium-power section. Note numerous alveoli (22), lumen (23), secretory granules (24) in glandular cells and basket cells (25). ×350

Fig. 17.3.(d)   Eye (monkey), low power, sagittal section. ×9

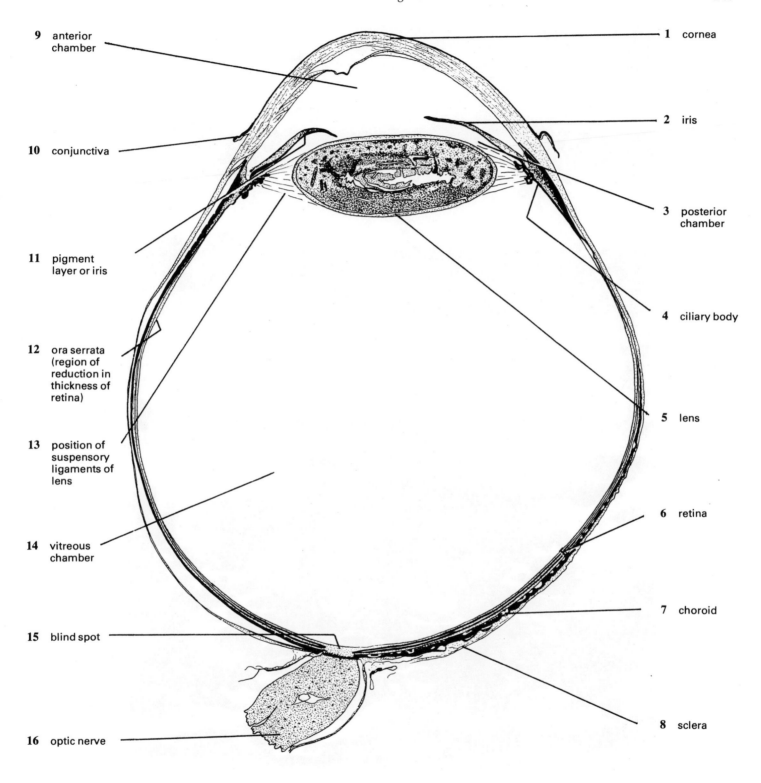

9 anterior chamber

10 conjunctiva

11 pigment layer or iris

12 ora serrata (region of reduction in thickness of retina)

13 position of suspensory ligaments of lens

14 vitreous chamber

15 blind spot

16 optic nerve

1 cornea

2 iris

3 posterior chamber

4 ciliary body

5 lens

6 retina

7 choroid

8 sclera

Fig. 17.3.(e)   Drawing of (d)

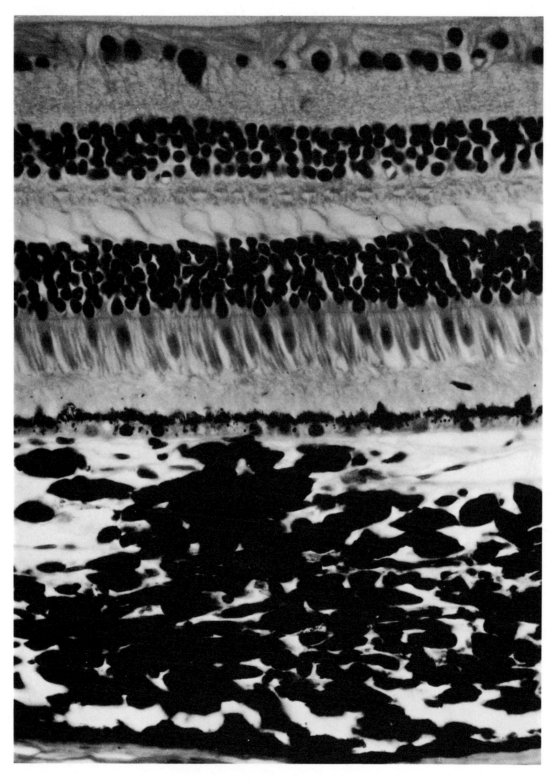

Fig. 17.4.(a)   Eye (monkey), medium-power section of retina. ×600.

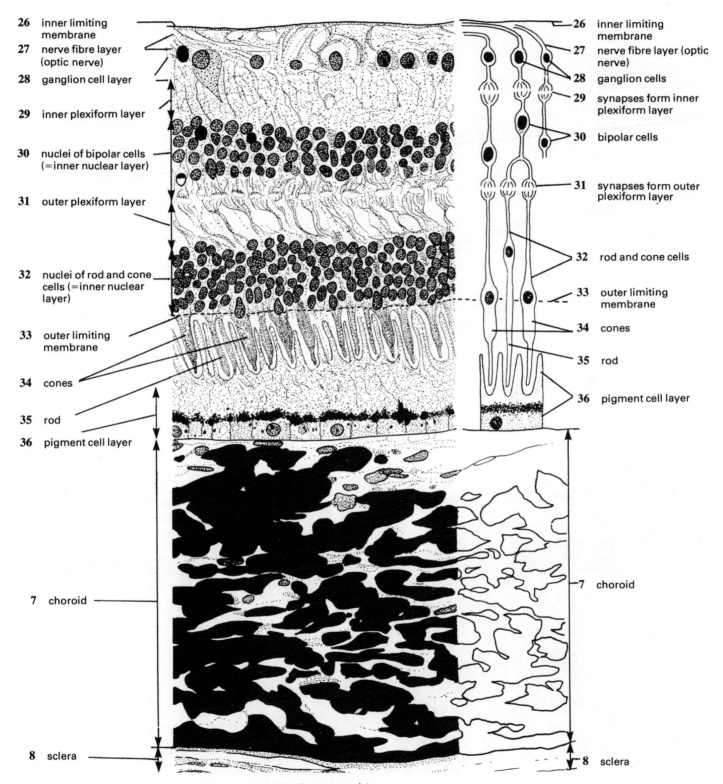

26 inner limiting membrane

27 nerve fibre layer (optic nerve)

28 ganglion cell layer

29 inner plexiform layer

30 nuclei of bipolar cells (=inner nuclear layer)

31 outer plexiform layer

32 nuclei of rod and cone cells (=inner nuclear layer)

33 outer limiting membrane

34 cones

35 rod

36 pigment cell layer

7 choroid

8 sclera

26 inner limiting membrane

27 nerve fibre layer (optic nerve)

28 ganglion cells

29 synapses form inner plexiform layer

30 bipolar cells

31 synapses form outer plexiform layer

32 rod and cone cells

33 outer limiting membrane

34 cones

35 rod

36 pigment cell layer

7 choroid

8 sclera

Fig. 17.4.(b)   Drawing of (a). (Upper right-hand side is diagrammatic).

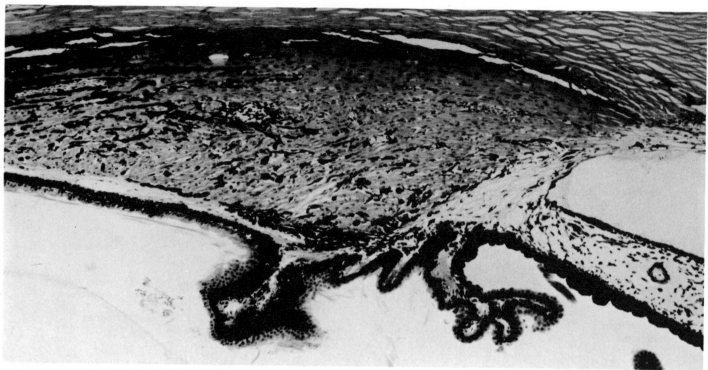

Fig. 17.5.(a)   Eye (monkey), medium-power section of ciliary body. ×120

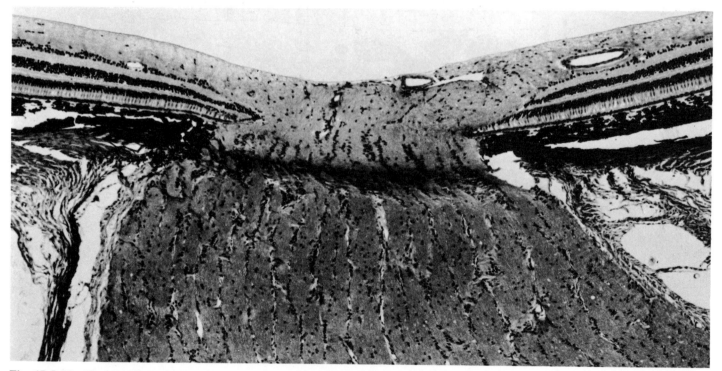

Fig. 17.5.(b)   Eye (monkey), medium-power section of entry of optic nerve (= blind spot). ×90

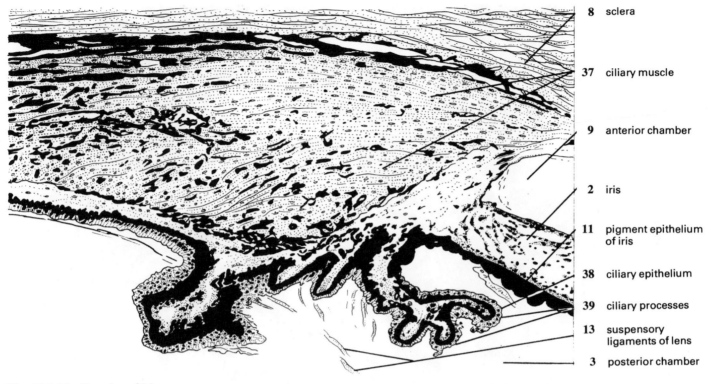

8 sclera

37 ciliary muscle

9 anterior chamber

2 iris

11 pigment epithelium of iris

38 ciliary epithelium

39 ciliary processes

13 suspensory ligaments of lens

3 posterior chamber

Fig. 17.5.(c) Drawing of (a)

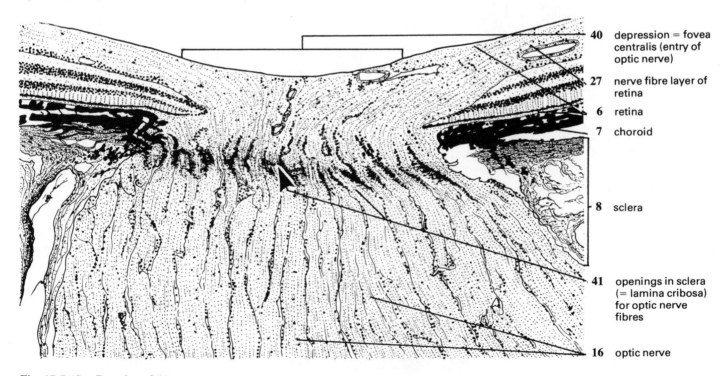

40 depression = fovea centralis (entry of optic nerve)

27 nerve fibre layer of retina

6 retina

7 choroid

8 sclera

41 openings in sclera (= lamina cribosa) for optic nerve fibres

16 optic nerve

Fig. 17.5.(d) Drawing of (b)

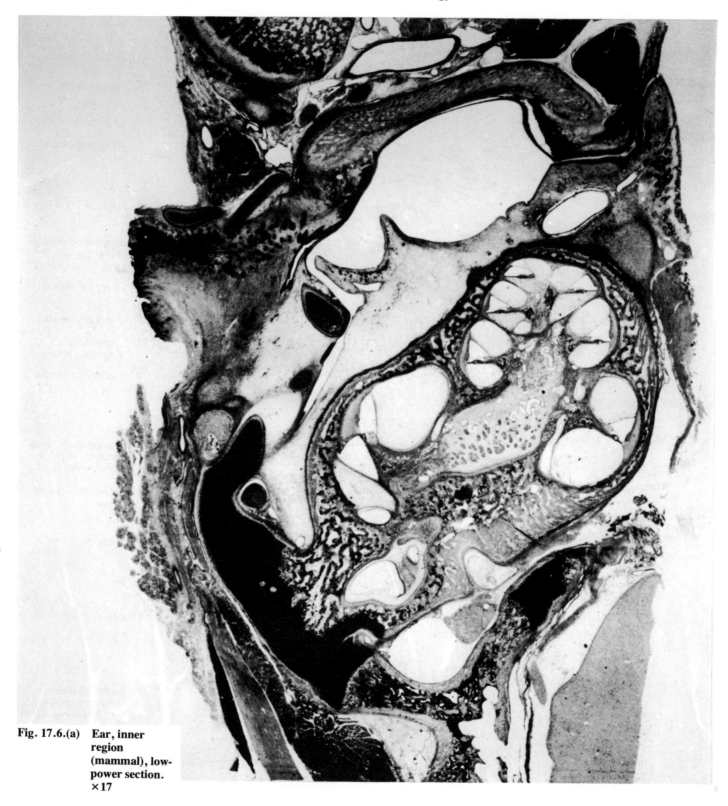

Fig. 17.6.(a) Ear, inner region (mammal), low-power section. ×17

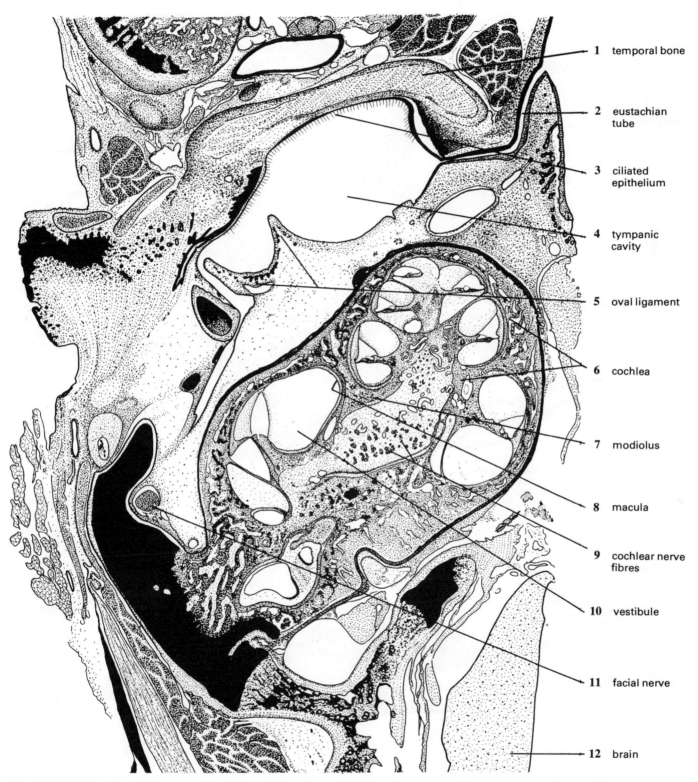

1	temporal bone
2	eustachian tube
3	ciliated epithelium
4	tympanic cavity
5	oval ligament
6	cochlea
7	modiolus
8	macula
9	cochlear nerve fibres
10	vestibule
11	facial nerve
12	brain

Fig. 17.6.(b) Drawing of (a)

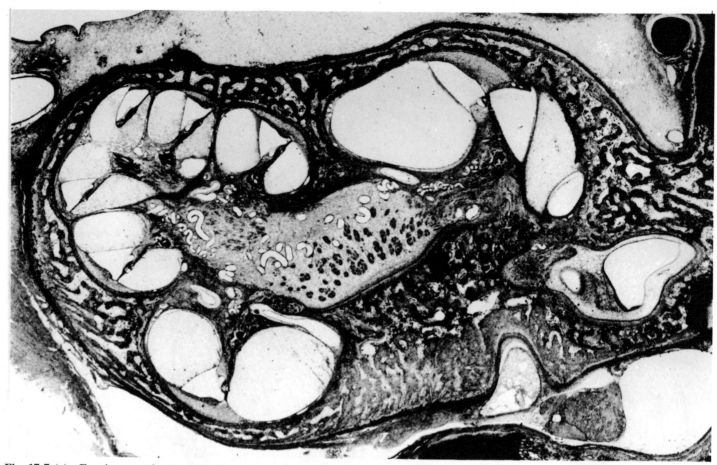

Fig. 17.7.(a)   Ear, inner region (mammal), medium-power section of cochlea. × 25

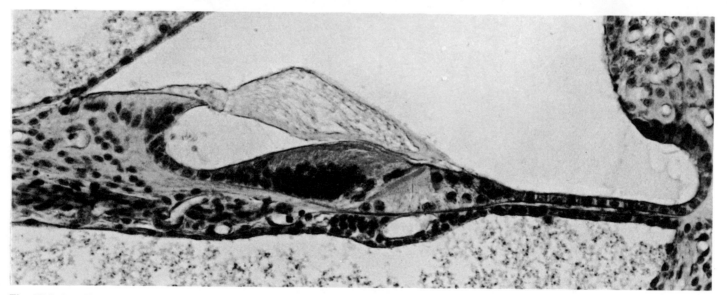

Fig. 17.7.(b)   Ear (mammal), high power showing details of organ of Corti. ×380

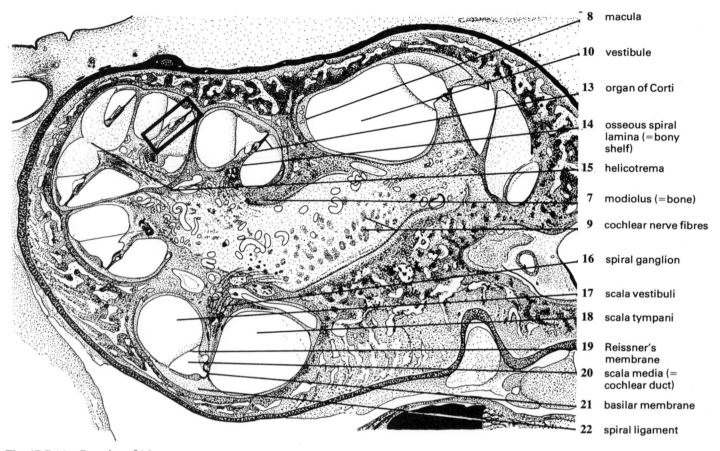

8   macula

10   vestibule

13   organ of Corti

14   osseous spiral lamina (=bony shelf)

15   helicotrema

7   modiolus (=bone)

9   cochlear nerve fibres

16   spiral ganglion

17   scala vestibuli

18   scala tympani

19   Reissner's membrane

20   scala media (= cochlear duct)

21   basilar membrane

22   spiral ligament

Fig. 17.7.(c)   Drawing of (a)

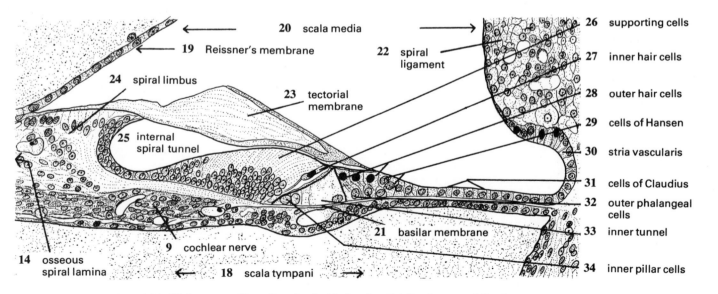

20   scala media

19   Reissner's membrane

22   spiral ligament

24   spiral limbus

23   tectorial membrane

25   internal spiral tunnel

26   supporting cells

27   inner hair cells

28   outer hair cells

29   cells of Hansen

30   stria vascularis

31   cells of Claudius

32   outer phalangeal cells

33   inner tunnel

34   inner pillar cells

9   cochlear nerve

14   osseous spiral lamina

21   basilar membrane

18   scala tympani

Fig. 17.7.(d)   Drawing of (b). High power of boxed region in (c) showing details of organ of Corti

Further Reading

Bloom, W. and Fawcett, D. W. (1968). *A Textbook of Histology,* 9th edn, W. B. Saunders, Philadelphia, London and Toronto.

Di Fiore, M. S. H. (1967). *Atlas of Human Histology,* 3rd edn, Henry Kimpton, London.

Freeman, W. H. and Bracegirdle, B. (1979). *An Advanced Atlas of Histology,* Heinemann Educational Books, London.

Glenister, T. W. A. and Ross, J. R. W. (1974). *Anatomy and Physiology for Nurses,* 2nd edn, William Heinemann Medical Books, London.

Ham, A. W. (1969). *Histology,* 6th edn, Lippincott, Philadelphia and Toronto.

McNaught, A. B. and Callander, R. (1975). *Illustrated Physiology,* 3rd edn, Churchill Livingstone, Edinburgh, London and New York.

Netter, F. H. (1970). *The CIBA Collection of Medical Illustrations,* vol. 4, *Endocrine System and Selected Metabolic Diseases,* CIBA Publications Dept.

Nonidez, J. F. and Windle, W. F. (1953). *Textbook of Histology,* 2nd edn, McGraw-Hill, New York, Toronto and London.

Reith, E. J. and Ross, M. H. (1970). *Atlas of Descriptive Histology,* 2nd edn, Harper & Row, London (now available as 3rd edn, 1977).

Rowett, H. G. Q. (1974). *The Rat as a Small Mammal,* 3rd edn, John Murray, London.

Index